I HAD COVID AND IT HURTS

Dealing with the loud silence

Rcurtis Fantpayne Jamerson

This book is dedicated to my Children and my grandchildren:

Daddysgirl Jamerson - Aleczandria Tyisha Jamerson my daughter. I'm so proud of my daughter and her accomplishments her parenting skills and her over-all attitude about life. About 8 years ago she opened an adult family home bought a condominium to rent and started a cleaning service. Since then, she got engaged to her Fiancé Sanareth and she's all happy. My daughter checked on me every day and I know you're probably thinking that's what's she supposed to do; no, obviously you didn't hear my description of Aleczandria Tyisha Jamerson. She is supposed to make sure her program is not distracted and pray for me knowing God's hand and his son Jesus precious blood is protecting me. She checks in on me every day and I can tell it is not easy for her to do with all the negative and unwelcome news out in social media. So, like I said "Daddysgirl" Jamerson make sure I hear from her every day. I love you to the moon past infinity to the next life babylove!

Atilio - My son, my twin, my talented gent. Atilio is a rock-star. Lives in sunny California, he's been in countless music videos, commercials, big events, he's directed, choreographed huge productions and he's a songwriter too. With all these goings on, you would think it'd be tough for him to reach out. Obviously, it's not because he does, and it makes me feel some-kind -of -special whenever he does. Keep it up son, enormously proud! Love you more than you can ever imagine!

Nai Nai and Geno - My grand babies, the reason I work, survive, and strive to make forward progress is for you two! Papa Deuces is proud as heck to be your grandpa! You two are so intelligent and smart, witty, strong minded, I love your leadership qualities in the making! You take your education seriously, you are obedient until you must be checked which is cool because you are not perfect, nor do we expect you to be. Your future is the brightest thing in your future so, make sure you take full advantage of that fact and get everything you got coming your way. You two, I don't know how not, to love, you are my proudest moments on a daily basis. Keep loving me as I love on you - "Deuces"

Special dedication to the love of the rest of my life:

Natasha -You saved my life, you caressed my life, you cuddled my life, you changed my life, you enhanced my life's happiness, you brought natural beauty into my life, you brought joy back into my life, you reminded me what the meaning of a beautiful life really means and oh how good it feels! You are the reason I limp and lean no more to the right because "my rib" is now whole again! Natasha Simona Sims I solemnly vow to keep you blushing as much as possible, satisfied with my forward progress, keep your spirits uplifted, keep your soul fed with divine foods from our father God in Heaven, you will never be thirsty or hungry for knowledge because it's a prayer away, they're will be no "angry bed", no bad energy carried over until the next day, "we as one" is our mantra and "we as one" will always be referred to it as our guide. Natasha, thank you for the kind, no nonsense, sweet "but will chip a tooth, if necessary," no fear, beautiful spirit and soul, honest, passionate, compassionate, loving woman that you only know how to be. My Germanchocolate Gigga! Baby, Love is God and God is Love and what I feel for you has not ever been said because words are simply not enough. Well let me try…. Natasha, not only do you complete me you make me complete, you are also 50% of my smile, half of my life, all my love and laughter and you are my everything I didn't even know a woman could be. I can't wait to make you Mrs. Natasha Simona Jamerson 4/22//2022 My love 4U is from the Heavens.

Thank you to the staff at Good Samaritan Hospital who kept me alive!

Dr Perez

Nurse Tara

Nurse Jackie

And the rest of the staff on the fifth and eighth floors!

God bless you all!

I dedicate this book to all the victims and their families who could not be with them during this bout with Covid.

Friends and family that I didn't mention, know that your prayers were heard and appreciated and I love you too.

Cover: ©THISIS4UPUBLISHING
Designed by Barbara Christensen, Be Light Create LLC
Photo Credits: Rcurtis Fantpayne Jamerson
Formatting: Barbara Christensen/Be Light Create LLC
Publishing: THISIS4UPUBLISHING Copyright © 2021

I Had Covid And It Hurts / Rcurtis Fantpayne Jamerson -- 1st ed.

AASD Publishing

ISBN   9798853506848

Contents

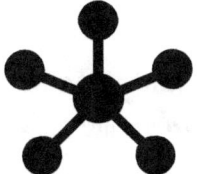

INTRODUCTION

T uesday August 17,2021 woke up got out of bed with my normal routine to get ready for work. Dropped and did 40 push-ups then got in the shower. When I got out I did another 40 push-ups. Then I put on my pants and did another 25. Then I got totally dressed got a sweet kiss on the way out the garage by my fiancé. It is sitting about 70 degrees already at 7:45am in the Emerald City. It is so beautiful!

Throughout the day I had this horrible headache that would come and go. I have never been much of a medicine type guy, more of a self-healer if you will. So, massaging my temples was an all-day task for me in between sales. Got off work stopped by my office to check the set-up for the "Thatguy Rcurtis Show" the name of my talk show previously titled "RnR Live Jamm Session Presents."

Still massaging my temples, and now I am feeling like I might have a fever. Since it had really been hot and uncomfortable sleeping at night in the Pacific Northwest, we slept with the fans blowing and the windows open which I attributed to my headache and fever. As I got a little worse, my energy level dropped. I spoke to my younger brother and he insisted I get tested for Covid. I didn't that night, but I did the next day, Thursday.

After our talk, I went to my office to set-up and do "Thatguy Rcurtis Show" but something did not feel quite right. I called my fiancé and explained to her what I was feeling, and she said to come after the show, and she would take care of me. I explained to her that I felt if I did not leave and go now, I was not going to make it until tomorrow.

I drove to her place and that saved my life. Had I stayed in my office I would have not known what to do and would have passed away in my sleep. I got there, did the show with minimal energy, but I got through it. Then it seemed that it was over. Fever, chills, headache, and diarrhea. I was a mess. I sent a text to my job to inform them of my condition and told them I took the Covid test should have results back in 48 hours (about 2 days). While waiting for my results I noticed my sense of taste disappeared. I then knew the test would more than likely come back positive. Meanwhile on the home-front the fiancé went into full natural path with a hint of traditional medicine on top. Vitamin this, cough syrup that, steam (face) baths. I mean if Natasha could have single-handedly saved me herself, she would have chosen to do so. And the road to recovery begins.

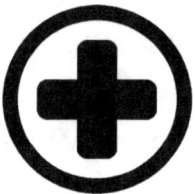

CHAPTER ONE

Ten o'clock in the evening, Sunday August 22,2021 Natasha called 911 as my blood pressure was deathly low. I'm feverish and in some pain, as well. Now, normally I would have just let her take me, but this was not a time to be thinking about me and my likes or dis-likes of hospitals and aid cars and all the hidden fees. This was time to be obedient and get in the damned EMT and get it to the hospital!

I remember thinking how long the ride was taking, and I didn't know where the hospital was in reference to my residence. I could hear the EMT saying, "We'll be there in 15." Man, that was the longest 15 minutes ever! Thoughts were parading all through my head. My brother saying no! Don't ever go to the hospital unless it's deathly necessary! I totally understand why he felt that way considering he had Covid, and he and my sister-in-law treated themselves in their home.

Well, I blew that by mistaking getting fresh air, for walking around the block a few times which is what I did and paid for it dearly! Coughing non-stop blood pressure dropping, temperature rising and head-ache throbbing. So let me take you back to the day before all these shenanigans.

Natasha had taken me to Multi-Care Clinic after the walking fiasco, and they checked me out and gave me an inhaler then sent me home. Fever was lower and since Natasha made me drink some "soup with my salt" my blood pressure raised up a lot higher, as well.

Natasha shared with me that when she was taking care of me post the clinic/hospital stay, she wasn't fearful, but instead wanted to ensure she was taking care of me as best as she could. She was in caretaker mode so to speak. It wasn't until she realized that my condition was getting worse and needed to be hospitalized that she became fearful that she would lose me. See, she had experienced the loss of a boyfriend before and she wasn't ready to go through that again. Seeing me helpless and so sick brought back painful memories for her.

Here's the short of it, Natasha was in a serious commitment with an amazing man we are going to call, Jeremy, and he was diagnosed with a form of cancer at the early age of 26. This is how wonderful this woman Natasha was, and is. She researched natural medicines that would not only help Jeremy, but practically cure him. They went to a naturopath, and then had him juicing, taking vitamins and making sure his meals were plant-based and most importantly, she kept him away from all sugar. Apparently, the sugar would provoke cancer activity.

Everything was going as planned, they were in a great place, the doctors on his team said his cancer had gone into remission and whatever he was doing, keep it up! Well, you know how we "hard heads" are. He did keep up the regimen; however, there was only one problem... he couldn't stay away from the sugar.

Natasha said she found all kinds of snicker wrappers and other candy that he was sneaking into their home. Apparently, Jeremy loved snicker bars and just couldn't stop eating them. So, just like anything that we allow to control us.... It took total control and eventually it (the snicker bars) consumed him, and his cancer came back even more aggressive than before and about eight months later he met his demise.

Natasha witnessed it all, watching him take his last breath. I can only imagine how she felt when I was barely responsive to the paramedics when they came to pick me up. There most definitely had to have been some fear of losing another boyfriend! You never would have known it though; she was on it! I could hear but I was unable to respond. I mean she was answering their questions without any hesitation, telling them what she administered to me before they arrived, what my blood pressure and my oxygen levels were, I mean on it! I don't think any other woman would have known what to do, I think they would have just panicked, and I would not have made it. I truly believe that, wholeheartedly!

Now, fast-forward to September 12th, 2021. I am now out of the hospital and her nursing and nurturing abilities kick –in full throttle!

Breakfast was like clockwork as soon as she got up for work, lunch around noon or so, dinner between 4:30-5pm and in between she made sure I was taking my blood thinner meds and steroids for my lungs. This incredible woman! It took six months for my recovery but, I am now better than I ever was! I guess sometimes your angels here on earth have to be revealed to you in the flesh.

Fast-forward back to the EMT drop -off. You know what I hate about the emergency room the worst? The wait. Well, I guess since I came via EMT I had a little seniority.

Before we move deeper into the story can we talk about the vaccine? Shall we? My first views on it were just based on how I felt personally. So, my whole take on it in a nutshell was based on this belief, why would I put something in my body that I don't want in my body? I don't even get a flu shot for that same reason. I only get sick once every three years! I was not having it! My uncle Stan tried to convince me in his bullish tough-love - type way. My mom with her not so subtle hints, my brother Derrick with his articles and fact-finding. I mean I know they were all coming at me with nothing but love and I love them that much more for it. I can be stubborn sometimes, ok, most times. I'll admit it. I just could not get that concept through my mind successfully.

You know what I hate about emergency rooms the worst? The wait! Well, I guess since I came via EMT I had a little seniority. It isn't what you hope for, but when you need it, you'll be grateful.

"Dispatch we're pulling in now." So, we finally arrive at the hospital and then Natasha shows up shortly thereafter. As aforementioned I felt as though I had some type of seniority due to the fact I arrived in the back of an EMT because they rushed me to triage oh wait..., now I'm in the hallway again so much for that seniority. Anyway, now the reason I'm in here is because we told them in the beginning, I have been diagnosed with Covid Natasha is here with me the whole time. They must give me a Covid test now.

The COVID test comes back positive, and Natasha is not allowed back in the room now because Covid patients can't have visitors. You know I'm hot! What do you mean she has been in here the whole time, and you already knew I had Covid that's not making any sense to me! Well sir, we had to do our own test and after our test came back positive it was conclusive. Now, you can leave if you want. What! Yes. I did not want to be here anyway and your attitude sucks lady! Natasha said, "No baby, you are here to get well." She looked at the lady and said, "He ain't going nowhere."

Then I had a Dr just sticking his head into the room for a second. You qualify for plasma transplant, but you could run the risk of acquiring aids or whatever the donor might have. No, not interested in that. There is also this medication that is not FDA approved yet if you want it, I could give it to you right now. No! Take the chance of being worse off than I am now….? Negative ghost rider! And then he just kept popping in and saying it randomly like the objective was not to help but to boost his sales for these wonder drugs. You're serious right now?

My mom who just recently conquered breast cancer is dealing with some non-FDA approved drug that her doctor convinced her to try. Not me Patna! I'm in God's unchanging hands. I can remember laying there damn near lifeless but never afraid. I was frustrated because I was unable to regulate my breathing and control my violent cough while trying to take a breath through my nose out my mouth felt like all I was doing was hyperventilating. Super freakin' frustrating for me. I just wanted to breathe on my own! I was all in my head now like, I can't catch my breath into panic mode, then suddenly I calmed down, caught my breath and was cool.

Wait a minute here comes the damned cough again! In through the nose out the mouth, in the nose out the mouth, in through the nose out the mouth dammit! It seemed like it was taking forever now the stress is kicking in along with some of the people I know and heard about who lost their lives in the hospital and not necessary from Covid but other simple things like a bump then find out that bump is actual stage four cancer and can't be treated. I mean all sorts of stuff goes through your head. In through your nose out your mouth close your eyes and concentrate, Rcurtis. Ok, better, there you go.

Now lay there and chill. Covid hurts. The pain while coughing, the headaches, the body shakes I mean all of it just hurts but guess what…. No pain, no gain and I for one was determined to gain my way up out of this without a doubt so, "help me Holy Ghost" every chance I got I reached for help from the heavens. Now, finally in comes another doctor with the news. "We're going to keep you overnight to keep an eye on you" when will I be out because my birthday is in two days, and I don't want to be here then. Really, you are not concerned about your birthday, and you are damn near on your deathbed. Stop -it! You were just saying something to make you feel like you are in control, you were not concerned about being out of here by your birthday you were really concerned about am I going to get out of here at all. Your birthday. Wow!

The Dr was like, "You'll be in here at least two or three days. This is a slow process, and we want to make sure you don't have to come back." Understood. I had to humble myself so that I could get into obedient patient mode. Obedient patient mode is very detrimental to your recovery. You must rely on these nurses and doctors to see you through and if you are a jerk patient.... Think about for a second there ain't no telling where you might end up. They are already short-staffed and now their careers are being threatened, there is no telling how many deaths they see in one day. So, now not only do they have to deal with you, they also have to locate some type of disconnect to not go batty and you think it is ok to be a jerk patient. Go ahead. Let me know how that works out for you. "You get more bees with honey than you do with shit" over-stand that and lock it into your mental data it will take further. So now they say we have a room for you on the 8th floor. Ok, let's go. Violent coughing repeatedly in through the nose out the mouth, in through the nose out the mouth, in through the nose out the mouth come on you had it down! In through the nose out the mouth! Man! Finally! Ok, I've got to figure out how to not cough. Coughing is good because it is getting rid of the flem in your lungs. Great!

We're rolling me up to the 8th floor room #832. We arrive and guess what? Yep, you guessed it, violent coughing, spitting, violent shaking, chest pain and of course headache. This right here is crazy! I believe they had me in a mask the first night. Anyway, I was so uncomfortable and now a little intimidated. I do not like hospitals in case you can't tell. Nevertheless, I knew it was important for me to be here and on my best behavior especially if I wanted to get out.

So, now I'm getting IV's and medications, breathing treatments, blood pressure checked, blood work, asked if I'm in any pain you know the regular gamut. I answer and now it's time to lay it down. There is an oxygen measure that I'm supposed to keep up to about 88 at least mine was down to like 84. Perfect reason to be concerned. So, here they go. "Try to breathe in your nose and out your mouth" yeah ok I'm thinking thats what I've been doing this whole time now with this air flowing through my nose I am choking like nobody's business trying to regulate my breathing and focus on getting my oxygen levels up.... bro I'm a mess. Well, they said that's enough of that and two days later. "We're taking you down to the ICU. There is a high-flow on that floor plus they will give you closer attention. We just want to make sure you're making forward progress" I'm thinking am I going to have a tube down my throat?

I was feeling threatened, that's when I first got to the 8th floor by my doctor. "If we can't get your oxygen levels up, I'm sticking a tube down your throat" I was like no you are not you'll be calling Natasha. Oh, you have somebody on file. It was like he was just on some this is what it is, and you can't do anything about it all aggressive and rude. I don't know what that behavior was about but, we got past it and became surprisingly good friends especially when he asked if he could pray for me. It was an enormously powerful and deep spirit soul penetrator! The Holy Spirit was strong in my room. I was so touched I shed a few joyful tears.

See, you never know and that's why you always give a person the benefit of the doubt and take it from there. If I would have held that misunderstanding against him, I never would have gotten that powerful prayer and who knows where my spirits would have been with me harboring something that's small. There is this position on your stomach called "Cronin " and it is just that laying on your stomach and allowing for your lungs to work more efficiently basically backwards but boy does it work wonders for your recovery! I'm telling you guys I paid attention to every little detail I could. I had so many nurses and respiratory experts along with doctors saying "if you want to get out of here make sure you sleep in the Cronin position as much as possible you will expedite your recovery." So, me, Cronin every night and sometime during the day as well. I was determined, determined, determined. I was getting up out of this hospital in better condition than when I came in here for sure! I had one nurse say that sleeping on my side would work too. Negative! So, back on my belly I went. That was the answer that's what got me out of ICU so expeditiously oh yeah and this breathing apparatus exercise thingy that they also said would help expand my lungs. I'll take that too please. Here we go on our way to a speedy recovery Rcurtis!

This is not going to be tasteful at all but let me tell y'all about this incredible relief. Ok, so since I had that high flow breathing hose in my nose the whole time in ICU, I noticed one time in my nose some super hard and long crust. I thought it was my hair growing wild but nope that was not it at all. It was blood coagulated inside my nostrils! What! Are you serious? Could someone have warned me about this and how to get it out because I'm not only contending with this forced air in my nostrils now, but I also find out that I'm fighting through these huge blood scabs in my nose as well. Man, I'm really dealing with some insaneness now! Ok, call the nurse and see if we can figure out how to get these out because I have tried to just force them out. Ring the nurse's button…. Yes, is there anything we can do about these blood scabs in my nose, I'm sure if they were gone, I would be able to breathe a lot clearer.? Yes, I can give you some warm towels and you can work them out that way. Did not work. Next night yes is there any way we could get these blood scabs out of my nose? Let me try to put some warm water in your machine and within the next hour or so you should be able to blow them right out your nose.

Eureka!!!! It worked. I'm breathing clear as a whistle not contending with the forced air and the blood scabs! I am a new man breathing like a normal human being. It allowed me to sleep way better and all that! My oxygen level immediately got lowered because I could breathe. Amazing the little things in life and death if you don't find a way to control them. Your breathing, your thoughts, your faith. Real talk though this Covid is real it's not playing it's designed to kill, still and destroy us at any cost so let's be cognizant of our fellow man, woman, and child. Mask up vaccinated or not, show you care about your fellow brother or sister because if you don't, something bad is going to happen to you and not right now or soon but eventually. And all you have to do is care.

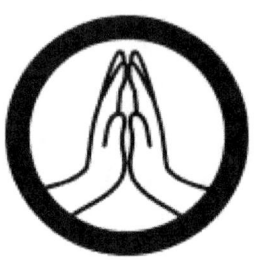

CHAPTER TWO

I am a true believer of God, his miracles, his love for me, and his concern for me. I appreciate all the gifts he's bestowed in me, and I just love him so much and I trust him with every inch of my life. When I'm in a mental dilemma and I need divine guidance, he knows and we talk in my quiet place in the wee hours of the morning 4:30, 5:30am. I love it because it gives him time to pour so much into me, I feel it immediately and oh you have never felt a satisfaction like receiving confirmation and more gifts at the same time! There is the gift of speaking in tongues (which I prayed for after I got jealous in church because I wanted it so badly; I received the gift the same day of prayer). I mean My God and I are having a glorious time! Then after my fulfillment I bless him in Jesus' name. Amen.

So, as far as my personal dilemma about the vaccine I would tell people, "When God tells me to take the vaccine it will already be in the works," And I meant that. Now I'm really wanting for answers because I really want to be obedient and safe around my family and love-ones I don't want to be the one who can't come around because I'm the carrier.

Ok, I'm going back to my quiet place. This time I specifically asked, "Will I be ok after this vaccine shot? " And I was told, "Don't worry I got you." So, what do I do immediately? I had Natasha schedule me an appointment for Pfizer that following Wednesday at the neighborhood Rite Aid. Now, check this out. Could not follow through with the appointment because of a fever I had developed 102. Back in bed and Natasha is now my caregiver and you know where my head is at right? That conversation had absolutely nothing to do with the vaccine that was all about me having Covid. And him letting me know that the road ahead is going to be rough, and he got me. So, don't panic. Wow! He is so awesome and wonderful. I'm glad he's my dad!

While waiting for the test results, I lose my sense of taste. The last thing I remember tasting was a PB&J sandwich after that... nothing. I could not smell my breath, or my under-arm alarm... nothing. That's when I knew the test would be positive. Un-like Jill Scott in her song "The Way" 4:30 can't wait to get home." 4:30 I could wait to get those results: positive.

Even though I figured as much it still hit hard. Covid! Really! Me! Mr. 150 push-ups a day? Mr. healthy! I know, a little over dramatic, but you gotta understand that's who I am, Mr. Everything in moderation. Mr. Positive, Mr. Blow a tree. Nevertheless, I am now a victim of this evil disease. Let me tell you something, it is so easy to get into your mental capacity and mess this thing up for yourself. I mean I would be choking and forget that it was my breath that I'm trying to catch, nurses and doctors just standing around while you are having a coughing fit, and nobody is moving toward you to help. Now, you are in your head like, am I going to die like this, I mean all the deaths go through your mind, people dying in the hospital without any love-ones around. It's a complete mess. I almost ran out of breath explaining that to you guys.

At the end of the day, if you don't have a great faith system, incredible friends and family support prayer warriors. You will meet your demise and to be honest you guys, even though these evil diseases are created by the evil one's disciples to kill as many human beings as possible.... I wholeheartedly believe not one of God's believers is supposed to die from Covid. Just know if it's evil we can't do it on our own; we are not as smart, strong, and we have not been on this earth long enough nor will we ever be. The Devil has been tormenting this earth for thousands of years and he is anxious to get this over with so he and his followers can finally take their rightful place in Hell. Stop taking credit that is not yours and grab some help that is always there for you whenever you want it. Back to my stay.

I didn't eat anything for four days before I got in the hospital and four more days while I was in the hospital. My stubborn self was, "I can't taste it anyway." It was not until one day in ICU this energetic nurse named Dennis came into my room, ripped open my curtains and demanded that I get up. Ok, that was random. It was cool though because it's exactly what I needed that day at that time and that precise moment. Dennis had me doing P/T before my schedule P/T he got me out of my funk and back to me. And, when he said, "You don't eat, you don't live" ding, ding, ding... that's all I needed to hear!

Living is very necessary for me to complete my journey and secure things for my grand babies not to mention the heavens dropped me off an angel to marry. So. I'm eating and drinking hospital food like it's the best tasting dish Ever! I'm lying; I had Natasha and my daughter Aleczandria bringing me food everyday.... lol. Funny, after that day I only saw Dennis from afar, he never came back to my room. Interesting Huh? Was this just his divine placement in my recovery? Whatever it was.... I'm grateful for his obedience.

Woke up this morning and looked over at the information board and it said, "He Loves God!" I knew who wrote it and I thanked her. She is great! Nurse Jackie. No, she is not like the one on TV, no drug addiction or anything like that, she is just a believer as well and a beautiful spirit. God bless her.

You never know where your words of wisdom can come from or specific words of encouragement directly for you. It's best to keep judgment out of the equation and live without prejudice or expectations. Honestly, if I had a narrow mind type attitude, I believe that negative energy would be very detrimental. And that can never be a good thing ever. What is the longest either of you have been admitted into the hospital wait, no visitors, just you and these Doctors and nurses to depend on for your recovery? Now, you can answer. I would venture to say out of 50 maybe 3 of you at best have been in longer than two weeks.

It's not fun and Covid hurts! The lack of control of your breathing, the pain in your chest from coughing violently, the mental stress and fear of being alone. It can really tear you down if you allow it to. Covid is real ladies and gentlemen it's not evincible though.

Faith, strong friends and family support crew and tremendous prayer warriors. You must be a devout believer though, or it's all for not. You're probably thinking, and I hope not, man he's really pushing this religion thing. That's not it at all I'm just doing my part and giving you options with great benefits! I'm not saying this will convince you, but it certainly convinced me back in 1988/89 or so. I forget where I was working at the time, but I had received a nice bonus and I decided to repay God with my tithes; the offering of a drum set for the church. All I can say is, after that I asked for something in confidence, and he delivered! I don't know how you'll look at that testimony, but just to let you know, I didn't do that for a kick-back, in fact I was stumbling on a few bills that month; bills handled! So, this and many more answered prayers is my reason I love my father God so much! He keeps me!

There is an energy that once you are up around it, you are stuck in an effective way. All individual energy is not meant for every individual, sometimes it's only "for you".

I, like so many other black children grew up without my maternal father around which enabled me to latch on to whoever my mom decided to be in a relationship with at the time. I was not aware of who I was, but I did have something deep inside of me that kept me. You see, back in my elementary years it was mandatory for you to go to Sunday school, church, bible study and sometimes vacation bible school (for kids in the summertime) and even though at that age you weren't interested in going you went or else... Now every now and again I'd be a little interested in what the preacher was talking about but most times.... I was asleep!

What I noticed later in my life and if I'm not mistaken, I believe an adult referenced it to me as well; when you're sleeping you can still hear the message because you're absorbing it through dreams and sub-consciousness. I don't know how much of this is true, it's just something that was given to me. I was introduced to the Bible and prayers at an early age, and I have always been an advocate of them both since I can remember. The stories always fascinated me in a way that I could see them in plain sight! Crazy huh?

The way I look at it is even though I had no maternal father looking out for me, teaching me, helping me, encouraging me, I had my heavenly father and I believe that is what has kept me alive, loving, spiritual, strong, creative and understanding. Without my father in heaven, I WOULD'VE BEEN AN ABSOLUTE MESS! I have a relationship with God. I am not religious. I believe religion is man-made, whereas we all have our own individual relationships with God. And that is why I say, "All individual energy is not meant for every individual, sometimes it's only for you." Make sure you contest this theory if you feel any type of confusion because I am not here to provoke a tug-of -war within your spirit, I am here to help in any way that I can.

CHAPTER THREE

Well, this energy is now mine to share for the rest of our days. How can I explain Natasha? Moved to the United States from Germany at the tender age of nineteen, made a way for herself and her daughter, purchased homes, sold homes and now is the leader of twelve employees. She is a caring woman with a tremendous amount of zeal ta-boot. Her infectious smile combined with her beautiful long locks captivate her winning personality and her passion for others. She has a sweet disposition but don't let the sweetness fool Ya…. She is no push-over and she is no easy win; she can throw hands as well and if that doesn't work, feet too. What man wants a pre -Madonna in his camp anyway? Certainly not me. I want a real woman with a back- bone and no fear and still be aware of how to be my woman. That's Natasha and I love her to pieces.

If it were not for her, not only quick thinking but her humbleness and willingness to reach out to my daughter, brothers, and anyone else she felt could offer her any suggestions, I might not be alive right now to draft this book. She acted immediately without hesitation: vitamin this, cough syrup that, steam (face) baths, oxygen reader (suggested by my daughter Aleczandria) blood pressure cuffs. I mean she was on it! That's rare, as most women in that situation would panic (in my humble opinion). That's a lot though, and unless we have been educated or at least trained we as men would panic too. So, for her to move past panic to care-giver mode was amazing!

They say, "if it ain't in you, it ain't coming out" and that is so true. I mean no truer statement has been made except for "it ain't on you, it's in you." I suppose they are both saying the same thing in diverse ways of expression. It's all good. She's a trooper, I mean God took this one straight from my side and after all this time she is back! Natasha, I love you baby! Has it ever felt so good to say it out your mouth to the person you love that you can't wait to say it repeatedly? It's like a crazy boy's crush on a cute girl. She is amazing! So, she will officially be my wife come 04/22/22. I cannot wait!

OH wait, you know the fastest way to a man's heart is his stomach well…. SHE CAN BURN! She fries this chicken that needs to be in a restaurant and not because I'm biased, I'm saying because it's facts! It's like a different type of batter and has an amazing flavor. Delectable! She can Barbecue a little in the words of Maxwell - "A lil Sumthin Sumthin" yep, she is the total package. Oh, I left that part out on purpose, and I know you know what I mean. That ain't your business period! She loves to dance, walk in the club, arms up and she is in Heaven. So adorable and when she smiles it's like the sun finds its way through the clouds just to enhance it.

Thank you, Natasha, for making that bold move to the United States or I don't know if we would have this opportunity. We do though, thank you. Blushing forever security and love will be my vow to you always. Love your future - Rcurtis Fantpayne Jamerson.

Even meeting Natasha was meant to be.

Natasha is an amazing human being that was able to stop me in my tracks while I was running a hundred miles an hour so-to-speak. When we met, I was in awe of her being, we had a great conversation, and the funny thing is it was about everything and not something or another thing. We couldn't stop smiling as we were talking to each other, and it just felt like this is where I was supposed to be at this precise moment and time. I just wanted to know who she is?

Everything about her to me was unique and interesting, and I still was oblivious! I guess I can attribute it to, I was in a place that I didn't want to be in a committed relationship considering I had just released one that was no longer necessary to continue for whatever reason which is not important right now. I'd rather continue talking about my "gift from God" my "handpicked" gift from God, Natasha! You know how if you don't know something then there's the knowing and not recognizing at the same time? This was that. I didn't know that I would betroth this beautiful creature let alone marry her! I did though, and it was a beautiful ceremony!

Now, let's talk a little bit about the naysayers shall we. First, they will only get maybe one or two sentences just because that's not the energy that should be displayed here. Ok, so most would say that the reason I married Natasha is because she took care of me during my bout with Covid and they'd be wrong as two left shoes! Although my queen did stop her life while I was suffering from this awful disease, I had already made mention of it to her before I had gotten sick. It went like this, "If you and I are still hanging out next year do you think you'd want to have my last name?" So, sort of a light-weight proposal I suppose.

All I know is I'm sooooooo thankful for August 26th, 2020! That's when my life changed, and I grew more stronger and wiser and aware as a man! I learned to be more patient as well as positive and faithful. My life has just begun as far as I am concerned. I have a home and "home is where the heart is" not the building, it's the relationship because you know you're always safe "at home" I am so safe and secure in Natasha's arms and care. Her love for me is something I was unaware of existing. I've discovered the emotion of "like" and I truly believe that if you like the person you're with it will last beyond any little or even big dilemma's, misunderstanding, he-say she-say crap, arguments, fights or anything else, because you actually know who you're with and you know what to expect from them whenever there is a little bump in the road you appreciate the bond and the vows. You are ok, with letting it go, you're ok with letting them have a little space. And you look forward to making up. I have a woman, it's like my missing rib has found its way back into my body where it belongs..., I'm tremendously thankful! That, ladies and gents is my Natasha!

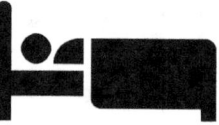

CHAPTER FOUR

My pride and joy is being able to say both my grand baby's birthdays are either on the day and the month or just the day of mine. There are synchronicities in life that are a part of the story. Geno, my little athlete, and scholar is on my birthday, August 25th and Nai Nai the sweetest soul you'll ever meet is May 25th. So, you see why I smile on a daily basis, it's an honor and a privilege to share those special days with my grand babies! I had BIG plans too. Jet skis cookouts are plenty fun. Had to cancel it all, because where your boy was, in the hospital on his born day. Geno enjoyed his cake though. A strawberry specialty cake! It looked so good! Aleczandria sent me some footage of the celebration.

I didn't mind being in the hospital on my born day especially when considering the alternative; right-side up in a coffin with my hands folded on my chest. Of course, my queen sent me the biggest Mylar balloon I'd ever seen and a beautiful heartfelt card. Could not see her though still that jester uplifted my spirits tremendously!

Not everybody knows how to pick out a greeting card. I learned from my mom, watching her go through every card until she found the perfect one saying what she would say. My mom, a provider, a very strong woman in her own rights, a friend to many people that she encounters.

My mom is like my Nana (may she rip) Nana was everybody's Nana. Liked and loved by all the children in the neighborhood, respected by all adults. And God fearing. The only thing my mom lacks in, to me, is communication skills with her children and grandchildren. My mother has no respect for her adult children which unfortunately has her going through things at this time that she wouldn't have if she respected her adult men that she raised and trusted that she did instill some good things in us that affords us the opportunity to help her. It's all good though, to a degree. See because of the lack of ability to communicate and the atmosphere of it all growing up, we also took on that burden with each other and it totally sucks! We must get our family love from other families because we don't know how to get along with each other either.

Now, don't get me wrong I mean we can hang out at times but when it comes to needing to talk about a situation that we could possibly help one another with, it's kept secret. What I mean by that is that one could know but, then you must be sworn to secrecy about it…. That is so dumb! You're only as good as your leader unless you recognize that is a trait you are not interested in continuing…. that's me! I refuse to keep that curse going, as a matter of fact I am praying and waiting for the opportune moment to bring my siblings together and discuss this horrible dark cloud over us! We must want to end it as a collective or it will trickle down to our children, grandchildren and so on.

My mother is at that age that either you change, or you stay the same and she's choosing to stay the same and I can respect that. I no longer get hurt behind trying to get my mom's approval (if you will) or figuring out a way to build a relationship with her that doesn't entail an argument or mistreatment (on her part) or anything like that. All in all, my mom is a good person who doesn't know it and is continuously trying to prove it instead of aging, growing and learning. I love my mom because she is my mom; however, it's impossible to like someone you don't know. In that knowing, I feel one of those tears trying to fall. It sucks not having a cool relationship with the woman who is responsible for you being on this earth!

I'm grateful I acquired that special greeting card gift from her, not to mention I am a poet and a songwriter and I suppose that helps a little. All throughout that day, I was getting the occasional aww, that's sad you got to spend your birthday in here, and I am like I'm good at least I'm alive. How quickly we forget to appreciate the simple things like "life". I never felt some type of way about being here for my birthday. I just focused on getting better and out of here. That is where my head was.

Just like jail this is not my permanent residence, a little extreme I know but that is how I feel about hospitals and incarceration they are supposed to be temporary not permanent. So, I refuse to get comfortable in either one.

Freedom and free-will is an awesome gift! And I don't know about you but when mine is threatened I take it really seriously. I have choices and with these choices there is either a benefit or a consequence, this is why I make my choices wisely. We all make mistakes and none of us are even close to perfect, we just get better with time if that is our individual choice.

I don't know if you've ever been incarcerated; I have, and it was uncomfortable for me. I wasn't going to make it comfortable either! It's something about being told what to do, when to do it, and where to do it that doesn't resonate with me. If I'm given free-will by the creator of this whole thing, then who has the right to force me to do anything? NOBODY, unless I made a choice to put me in a position or a circumstance to be with individuals who have been given that authority. And regardless of how big the alleged crime is or was, it will still put you in that "slave" position and under the control of a "master!" THINK, THINK AGAIN AND THINK ABOUT WHAT YOU JUST THOUGHT ABOUT THEN, MAKE A DECISION!

On another note, small mindedness is another form of incarceration (to me) when you think small you receive small results. Why not ask for what you want and then work towards achieving it, don't you deserve whatever is meant for you? People, we are not on this earth to suffer, hurt, beg, be lonely, be mistreated or any other negative attribute. We are all Gods' children and this whole thing belongs to him so we can have whatever it is we want! Ask and you shall receive those are his words through whomever he chose to send them through to get to us. Once we tap into our strengths and powers through our "relationship", there is literally no stopping us! This opens us to the relationships around us in a greater capacity, too.

Nai Nai texted me to check on me about every other day or so. Geno -not! I should turn his phone off! Just kidding, he's cool playing football and studying in two curricula, Mercer middle school and Rainier Scholars, so, you see he's a busy young man. Nai Nai, just started high school this year and I hate that I could not be there the first day! Oh well, we are raising some leaders and trend setters not followers, so I'm not worried; ok a little. That is my Nai Nai though. Ok get over it Papa Deuces and get yourself well.

Plenty of time to intimidate them little boys. Right, right, right. Plenty of time. I mean not to scare them too much but just to let them know who they got to go through. I was one of those little boys and I loved pretty girls, but I was shy and didn't come into myself until years later. Different times and eras though for me we had underage clubs to go to and house parties and some more stuff. We had buses that would run all night and we traveled in packs. My grand babies will not have that luxury, not with the way these kids think it's ok to pull a trigger and kill for no good reason.

You do know we are to blame for their behavior and attitude toward life's value. We had the opportunity to explain that the music you are listening to is strictly for entertainment, not a life's guide on how to live and survive. As musicians you had one job! One job! And you couldn't even do that right! Why would you endorse killing another black man regardless of what he's done to you, and minus if he did something to your family. Why??!! If you are that angry, put on some boxing gloves and go head-to-head until you're both tired. Then guess what? You both win, because neither one of you dies! Then we can be more powerful as a nation and as a people we need your young strong black man to carry the torch to our real freedom and prosperity.

Modern day slavery is just like Covid, and it's designed to control you just like Covid and if you let it, it will have its way with you just like Covid! I'm speaking out and up for mine..., STOP KILLING EACH OTHER GET TO KNOW ONE ANOTHER! How do you think we all met in the first place? More than likely, it was an altercation that got handled and passed. I will not let you kill my grand babies, and my grand babies are your ages, and my nieces and nephews are your age, you are my grand babies, nieces and nephews, so I love you all and I need you to dig deep within your soul and pull out that little boy who wishes his daddy loved him or his mom was not on drugs, or he or she never got molested by a relative or whatever it is. It's not your fight, it's not your battle it belongs to God! Your wounds have been already healed by the blood of Jesus the Christ, when he died on the cross. How many times does he have to die to prove it to you? Put your guns away and if you really want to have a gun and insist on killing ... join the military and be rewarded and decorated and get some pay for education for it. I'm just saying you are wasting your life and if you have children already, you are destroying them on a daily basis and they deserve much more than that..., BLACK MAN!

Make an unselfish decision, one time in your life.... any dummy can pull a trigger..., dummy!

YOU WILL NOT KILL MINE AND HOPEFULLY YOU WILL NOT KILL ANYMORE UNLESS YOU ENLIST IN THE MILITARY. I love you!

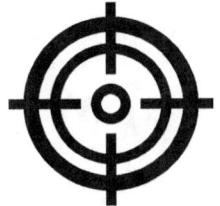

CHAPTER FIVE

Whew!! That last page took a lot out of me because I felt every word every death every cowardly move made, every bullet rattled, every drug the shooter or shooters were on while they sprayed an array of bullets, not caring who they hit, every fallen baby, every parent's cry, every arrogant attitude, every smug look on a police officer's face as to say, "and they're talking about us killing them!" Every confused perplexed emotion the shooters have in their spirits, every thought thereafter, every lost appetite due to the fear of now..., who's coming after me. Afterwards I thought, "what did I just do?" And it hurts like Covid.

These are children killing children!! How does that even happen???

Oh yeah, now I remember, children got rights and were entitled to call the police on their parents and then that turned into an effortless way to get away with quite a bit of grown-up behavior. Sex, drugs, drinking amongst other things they could get away with at the tender age of twelve and up. Remember that? The freaking world had parents scared and intimidated by their own kids. Teachers feared them, teachers were sleeping with them, then the students would come back and kill the bullies. I'm off this, for now. It's really making me angry right now and that's not good for my recovery.

How come it's not evident most times when we're dealing with our mistakes, how this is what we the people have done to ourselves? Case and point, we used to "pledge allegiance to the flag" now it wasn't the pledge, it was the unity involved that was healthy for us as children and it also made us feel good about something. Now, there is no pledge and no prayer, so we've told God that we got our schools, and we don't need him for that, we'll let him know when we need him. Since he doesn't force himself on us, he's like, "ok" you know where I'll be. Now we have elementary school kids' shooting's, grown women and men screwing Jr high school and high school children, it's a mess!

What do you think is going to happen if you get rid of your protection? The demons are going to have a field day, and we will have "hell on earth" as we do right now. Let me say this, I'm for, "to each his or her own" without a doubt. I mean both my children are in the LGBTQ community and I love them both dearly. What I'm not for is the demands and the expectations. Here's why I'm saying what I'm saying, and I had this conversation with my son Atilio. Your community and lifestyle are new to the world because before it was just what folk did and there were no demands or anything just living their lives and staying in their lane.

Now, think about this if you can indulge me for a few. The black race has been attempting to get certain rights and demands for 100's and 100's of years and the LGBTQ community has caught up and surpassed us by a long shot, congratulations! It seems just like everyone else on this earth you want more and more. That's wrong, I just want you to realize that your "race / community" is now the new minority and things are going to be a little difficult and the road is not going to be easy nor is it going to just be accepted the way you want it to be. People are mean, rude, evil, disrespectful, cruel and ignorant at times so since that is the case you must be more patient and deal with the reality that even though it's been a few years now, it's still new to the world and it more than likely will always be. No one has the right to dis-respect, mis-treat, hurt or harm anyone else because of how they choose to live their life, but they still do it, just the other day a friend of mine got called a "nigger" when he was attempting to apologize to the gentleman because he didn't see him on the road. So instead of getting that apology he lost his job that day due to my friends' level headedness, and his decision to take the issue to the guy's boss (owner of the company) who happened to be a minority as well.

We are all in this together and we must respect each other and love each other; life is too short for all the other bullshit! Facts! Anyway, I hope I didn't offend anyone. Honestly, I'm just talking to whoever is listening and I'm attempting to be very open as well as a "tad bit" diplomatic with my delivery. Afterall, "I did have covid, and it did hurt."

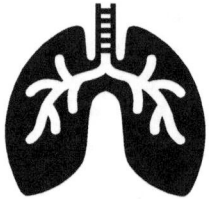

CHAPTER SIX

You know what? It's crazy the things that go through your mind when you have time to collect your thoughts.

Laying up in this hospital bed is allowing for just that. It's about 5:05 am and I'm up. The nurse just gave me a breathing treatment and checked my vitals which have been consistent for seven days (Praise God!) Some of you are thinking that if your vitals are good then you should be good. Negative Kemosabe, my lungs took a serious beatdown and along with the Covid, I had pneumonia and something going on with my kidneys. Covid is a challenge, and they must be thorough with me. I'm not out of the woods just yet, but I am getting there. It started me thinking, anyway, people are on a trip, "Well allow me to retort" - Samuel L Jackson "Pulp Fiction."

I have had "Thatguy Rcurtis Show " on a platform that I was asked to be on by the station director who I've known for at least thirty years. Imagine that he has not made one phone call or text to check up on me the whole time I've been down. Now, he's not like my "ace boon" no, but decency is decency, and nobody is that busy. Anyway, my show is on his platform, and it is now time to part ways. There are things about confidence and triumph that Covid has to teach us. I believe I've gotten what I need to be successful on my own. Too many times my show has started late without any communication from the engineer; very unprofessional and inconsiderate. He also has a show on the platform. Guess how many times his show gets started late? None!

The sad part about the folk in your hometown, is that most times there is some level of jealousy that you must deal with no matter what. I don't understand it not one bit! When I used to have performances, I would always scour the crowd to see if I recognized someone who could play an instrument or sang, and I would put them on stage and praise their performance, that's just me and who I am. I was told not to do that, because of up staging and silly things of that nature. It didn't matter to me, if you could get a gig, off mine, "congratulations!" I put a lot of money in a lot of these musicians and vocalist pockets. No one ever worked for me and made less than 100 dollars unless it was like a 20-minute gig or something then they still made a min of 75 dollars. Being a musician vocalist performer myself I could not see any other way.

This platform I am talking about I believe should be a lot more active in educating the show on how to become successful after leaving and more hands-on since it is receiving city and state monies and grants allegedly. I'm not throwing shade, just extremely disappointed in them is all. If you have been in the radio business for 30 plus years you should have so much more to give and give it! Everybody is not cut from the same cloth; some are blends instead of 100 % fabric. Whatever! Meanwhile, I am making plans to leave and go out on my own and be remarkably successful and if anyone wants to follow....

let's go! "Who's coming with me? "- Tom Cruise "Jerry Maguire"

Man, I was so angry yesterday, I had to calm down before I got my butt back in ICU…, besides Lil Homie had it under control but, simple things that should have not gone wrong did go wrong. We ask all our guest to check 15 minutes before show time, to make sure there are no technical difficulties and, if there are, then we should be able to get them ironed out before show begins; however, if the station engineer is running late without any communication, it will not work; it absolutely will not work! So, I'm out!

I have big plans and a whole new concept with a lot more goodies. I want a real live talk show! With the stage, band, guest stage, hype person for the crowd, and the whole thing. Guess what, I will have just that! Watch me as I grow! All I want to be is a blessing every day of my life, on the job and wherever else. I'm at the age that you don't try no more, you either do, or you don't. Decide and stick with it! Man, this birthday could have been my last. There was a possibility of me not making it these 365 days (about 12 months). But…, God said no!

So, since I'm still here..., obviously I have a purpose. Time to blow out that candle, now that I have the breath. It is time to get to work. Advocating for Covid, volunteering at the hospital, and being active with the mask -up mandate. People don't realize or just don't care that their mask is, for us, not them; vaccinated or not. Selfishness will kill us all! I will be doing my part in helping the cause.

Random: how come with all the moguls, billionaires, millionaires, and hundred thousandaires we still have a homeless problem in America? Home of the brave, land of the free! Makes no sense to me. Now, if I'm being honest there are a few homeless that I've talked to, and they said they'd rather live like they are living instead of how we are living and said we have way too much stress. Wow! Take a chance on the streets then deal with our everyday lives. That's Deep! I wake up every morning and write in this book and I never know where it is going to end up but, as the journey begins, I love it! I feel it, every word, sentence, paragraph, and page. This Covid is a real people, and it hurts! That which does not kill us, makes us stronger!!!

Can you envision being alone for a whole month with only your thoughts, voices, memories, issues, forthcomings, plans, fears, and strangers, but no family, or loved ones? It's just like being in solitary confinement and although I've been in solitary confinement, I can tell you I don't think I would survive it! and I also have to have my freedom to be likable.

Well in this case I was free to peruse my mind as I deemed necessary, and boy did I!

So-in-so just died last week from covid, am I going to die in this hospital?

Somebody just died today from this, am I going to wake up tomorrow?

They keep threatening to put on the ventilator, I don't want to be in an induced coma!

I can't wait to get out of here! I need to shave and cut my hair, how come me and my mom can't get it right? What the hell is wrong with me and my siblings!

What am I going to do when I get out? They say I'm going to need a portable oxygen tank when I get out of this hospital - I won't keep that one week, I promise you that!

I will be out of here for my birthday! Will I be out of here for my birthday? Damn! I hate that I can't breathe on my own!

Being in here sucks! I hate hospitals! I hope I don't have to go up to the 8th floor... oh, shit! They're taking me to the 8th floor! I gotta hurry up and get off this 8th floor! Do whatever they say to do, hurry up and get better!

That was a cool nurse, what the hell is wrong with that Doctor, who the hell does he think he's talking to?!?! Man, she's gotta have a lot of tattoos, she must be atheist. Oh wow! She wrote "he loves God on my patient board!" Don't judge a book by its cover, ever!

I miss my grandbabies!

How am I going to pay rent? My car payment is due, I gotta pay on my personal loan, how many people did I infect with this "evil ass" disease!!! and so on, and so on....

Your brain is all over the place and your thoughts are uber vulnerable, you are literally in the hands of the Doctors and nurses in-charge for eight hours at a time, then here comes the other shift for another eight hours. You have to be prayed up and ready to be the best patient EVER because not only are you going through this process, but these total strangers are also going through it with you and the thousands of other patients they have to care for, while living their own personal lives outside of saving lives and losing lives in the process. So, if you're an asshole and a jerk to deal with..., at any given time during this process either one of these delicate "guardian angels" can snap and end you! That is why it is important to always stay in your lane, you never know what someone is going through, where their threshold is and where it isn't!

People are unpredictable and rightfully so – no one person owes any other person anything and no one has to put up with "your or mines" ignorance or meanness either. So, think about that the next time you feel entitled or validated in your horrible behavior or better yet the next time you get slapped - up for your tongue!

We must make a better family; we must create a new trajectory for our future; kids and great grandkids - give them a chance to write their own story that has everything to do with why it's so much more peaceful and together... I don't know, I believe there is that possibility, I truly believe we have it in us. Wouldn't it be better and make you feel like you've made an impact in this lifetime, if we were to witness some dramatic change in how we treated each other as a "people" not just a race of people but as God intended for us to be "as one" people? Don't you think that once your work is done on this planet and it is good, you'd transition to the next "whatever" with a HUGE smile in your whole spirit and soul?

That's what I want. I don't want to wonder if I changed this or did this, or even followed through with... What would've happened? I want to be sure that I did all I could, and some worked and some failed, but I attempted! Does that make sense to you? I hope so.

We all have a "soul partner" within us. What I mean by that is that when we hear "common sense" speaking that is our "soul partner" attempting to guide us on our path keeping us off of others' trails; we don't always listen though and that's when we fall down. We don't stay down though as long as we reach our hand up to be grabbed by our "soul partner" then we get back on our way to our path. When we wake up in the morning it's a new day, this is when we must make a decision to make it better than it was yesterday. Why? I don't know, I thought maybe you could tell me. PONDER THAT FOR A FEW. It's not a test, it is a testament though. Hmmmh. I had to chuckle at that, just because. Do you use your "common sense?" Have you ever questioned that, or do you just take for granted that you have "common sense" so you're obviously using it? First of all, if this is the way you feel, then you're a little arrogant, secondly, we should take absolutely nothing or no one for granted! Period! Although we do have free will, we still must be considerate of all that exists and all that is within. That's just (in) my opinion.

You know what? I've come to realize that "LIFE" is not as complicated as we make it, it's actually pretty darn simple as long as you follow your path that was designed for you. Now, don't get me wrong we will have some stumbling blocks along the way that we will actually fall over and have to figure out how to recover from but, all in all it's all about the relationship we have with our superior being, our savior, our "great I AM" our higher power, our go-to or less. Think about it, when you awake in the morning do you carry over or begin anew, do you try to fix yesterday or do discover a break-through, are you already in defense mode or are you ready to conquer, are you still complaining or are you thriving to accomplish a goal (today)? Just those simple little details can create a whole new atmosphere for you to enjoy a better life experience.

Take it from a fella who has survived "one hundred percent oxygen" encounters. I don't think I've ever enjoyed my life as much as I am right now! THANK YOU, JESUS! HALLELUJAH! I'M ALIVE!

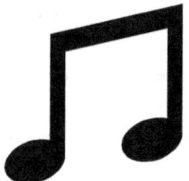

CHAPTER SEVEN

Here lately I've been on my R&B music here for my slumber. I noticed something about Anthony Hamilton. He bases a lot of his songs about his women cheating on him with his friends. That's crazy! Powerful lyrics! And the music and his background vocalist are phenomenal! Bruh, damn all your songs are about cheating girlfriends? Then

Raheem DeVaughn is always talking about smashing all the time. No judging, but one extreme to the next of nothing. Our gifts are given to us to give back in a way that someone will be edified and made whole again. We humans are too much sometimes but it is all good.

I also noticed Luther Vandross singing a little closer. He had a lot of dramatics and theatrical acrobatics with his performances and a lot of controlled breathing, he'd hold back when he needed to take it down some octaves and he would always slowly bring up to a range he knew he could hit undoubtedly. He didn't take any chances of cracking, he was very precise and on point. Singers are extremely nervous and always on blast so, we must always have a plan of action and if we are singing ill, it is so important, we stay in a range that we can play around with comfortably. I've had that happen a few times and felt like my performance was sub-par. And after the show there was always someone approaching with, "I have never heard you perform like that" and was told by many in the crowd that is the best I've heard you sing in a long time. The crazy thing about it is, if I had to duplicate it, I would not know what to do because I was working around the music and doing all kinds of acrobatics with my vocals, avoiding any cracks or that whisper, and whatever it took not to sound horrible.

I love singing though, it has been a passion since I can remember. I'd be in the mirror mimicking "The Jackson 5" . I had my make-believe audience. I would like to thank the folks for coming out. Kids and our imaginations, right? Too bad they don't get to use those these days. I remember one day at work helping a client and her 6-year-old daughter said, "mommy since I've been so good this whole time, can I get an app?" I said did she just ask you for an app? She said yes, she did. I said man, times have changed from, mommy can we go to the toy store or mommy can we get some ice cream to mommy can I have an app; red light green light is all the way out the picture. What about interaction? Wait, they can do that all around the world now.

Music is the universal language, the heartbeat of our lives, and the sound prints to our struggles. It's kept me sane up here. I sleep on it, and it wakes me up feeling alive and free. From jazz to r&b. I just realized, I have not listened to any rap, old school or new. Interesting..., It just is not the type of energy I need now while healing, I need chill real music from the soul. No offense. Just not feeling the arrogant, twerky (obviously not a word) proud type of behavior at all honestly.

We need change in every aspect of that word change. Change the attitude, change the expectation of us as Individuals, change in every community, change the school system back to prayer in the classroom , change the school curriculum so that it is more fair to all races creeds and religions, change incarcerations to rehabilitations and enlistations (made up word) to the military, change the ok for a police officer to kill another black, brown man or woman in cold blood and have it justified by I felt threatened because that is utter BULLSHIT!!! How do you feel threatened when they have a wallet, and you have a gun!!?? Stop-it!!! Change is very necessary not now but right now! So, do your part!

Musicians, you have a responsibility to these young people buying your music and idolizing you. Remember, God is a jealous God and after all he does for us, he reserves the right to be just that! Don't get caught up in that wrath. Unless you have already sold your soul to the enemy which I believe the lot of you have done you better change your algorithm. Today, I heard the best quote on a song I've never heard from an artist I didn't know existed. Adrian Bagher - "If you want to leave me, go ahead and go on. See I'm a good man baby; good men don't stay single long" One of the most powerful statements made, and true.

See, I try to gather information from wherever I can, to better my understanding while I journey this planet. For example, I will never forget, about age 15 or 16 my dad and I were on our way out the door at the same time, so I asked if he was going my way and he said yes. Cool, I thought. About halfway there, I was filling a nice little bond and decided to be all grown and cordial and I offered pops some gas money. Check out his response; my daddy told me, "if I turn down money, I won't ever have none" and he took that 20-dollar bill and put it right in his pocket.

Now, what are you guys thinking I'm curious...? Was he wrong for taking my money or was there a lesson there? This day, I say, a lesson, that day I was devastated, because I really thought I was going to hear, don't worry about it son I'm going that way anyway. Tough love, huh? Anyway, the lesson was don't have any expectations and no one owes you anything not even your parents. Think about it, he didn't owe me the ride and even though he explained why he was taking my money he did give me his bullshit reason. The reason I call bullshit is because he didn't even talk to his father.... Lol! The lesson was learned though. Big C – RIH.

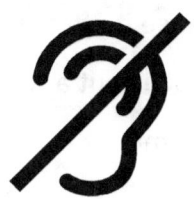

CHAPTER EIGHT

My mom moved out of my dad's house and bought a house down the street that she still resides in. This is my dad, who I considered to be "my dad" due to my biological father being in- present. Lesson? Absolutely!!!

My mom was a straight up boss for that move, I still stress that to her to this very day. I'm leaving you and I'm not going to my parents or a relative nor a friend NOPE I'm moving down the block to my new home and I'm buying a brand-new car! That's when you have that relationship with God, and you know it. My mommy is a pillar of strength and determination. They say you are wise when you learn from others' mistakes instead of your own because it affords you the opportunity not to make those same mistakes but a whole mess of others instead. It Makes sense to me.

I learned a lot from being in this hospital, like patience, keeping my mouth closed unless there is a question being posed to me or I would indirectly be disrespectful because of my common sense kicking in when it is time for me to shut up! See not all these nurses are efficient, attentive, loving, or caring and it is ok because they still must do their basic duties and that's all you need from them anyway.

Focus on what's positive, not negative. It will make for a better day and wish whoever is in your room at that time a great and blessed day and watch how yours turns out.

Take your time, don't rush anything and question everything. Do all the silly exercises and treatments I mean do it all and pay attention to the details of the instructions. I had to calm down because I wanted out of here so bad. Understand you are not here but because it was your turn in the lottery. IT'S BECAUSE YOU'RE REALLY ILL!!! And the only way you are going to get better is to be a humble and obedient patient otherwise you might not make it my friend. I came in here not looking good at all and now I'm at 6% oxygen instead of 100% and that's from realizing it is not my fight it is my responsibility to get well. I would not wish this on my worst enemy (if I had any) I am so serious! This is not cool by any stretch of the imagination, you guys. I hope none of you ever get Covid, it hurts.

Dry coughs are the worst but very necessary and important for your lungs to expand and allow for more breathing capacity. While lying in my bed I notice little details like the water in the machine to keep my nose from stinging, the settled flow of air coming through the apparatus on my face to help me breathe.

Then there is the silence. No noise, no interruptions, no responsibilities, no dos or don'ts, no rhyme or reason, just silence. The cool thing about silence is that it has no rules, or guidelines, it just is silence all by itself. So, what I do with it is appreciate and respect it enough to share with it and it works out swell. Like, I put positive energy into it just to make sure we start the day off right. Another thing is I am thankful for it.

Anything or anybody you show appreciation is going to be extra nice to you and make sure you have what you need. Can't really do too much singing in my current condition but normally I would serenade it with a nice tune. Silence is golden this is what they say (I have yet to know who they are) anyway at the end of the day.... It is very precious to our lives. With silence you are vulnerable. You must deal with you, entertain you, enjoy and get to know you. There is no other way around it but through you. How important is that? Hanging out with you. I had an ex-years ago that would just show up at my house to make sure I didn't have another woman over my house just because I said I want to and hang at my place for a while. And that was it, I wanted to be in my space to collect my thoughts or catch-up with or whatever, but she didn't get that.

She'd go through my closets, under the bed I mean she was so silly I had to laugh and then explain to her no, I just wanted to come home for a while.... We're good. Then soon after too many of those episodes she had to be dismissed before I got hurt. Coo, coo coo, coo for Cocoa puffs. Gotta go!

Sitting up in this hospital going through this terribly slow process of recovering really has me thinking about a lot of things that I can do to try to make a difference in our community and abroad. I plan on volunteering at this hospital and then maybe more. I want to be a speaker on this Covid monster. I want to try to help more people to want to live and not give into their confused mind state. I want to be part of their support system that says, you can do this, don't give up, "God got you!" No one is supposed to die from this evil man-made disease. It is just another trick of the adversary to get in your head and take full control and then kill you. Your faith system is in your bloodline. I'm not the most educated on this disease in fact I'm not educated on it at all but, I'm going through it and I'm experiencing the good, bad, and ugly of it all so. I guess I can call myself somewhat of an expert on this Covid virus considering.

Yeah, silence is golden, and I love it because it motivated me to draft this book and really hope this can help at least one person then it is not in vain.

CHAPTER NINE

'm meeting a lot of new career nurses for the last few days. I oftentimes would ask how they feel about what they do and how they felt about the mask mandate and also the new vaccine weight on them about losing their job if they are not vaccinated. One said, "Well, I'm using my religion to try to get out of it but, the union said that's not going to really work"

While another replied, "I don't know how to feel about it because I'm new in the field and I need to be protected and I also want to protect my patients. Hell, the vaccine isn't even proven to be full-proof, you can still get Covid and pass it along and there is no documented proof that these vaccines do work. As a matter of fact, the vaccine is temporary; six months I believe." This one said, "I'll just cross that bridge when I get to it." See, look at some of you already judging. You can't judge these nurses, their threat to their lively-hood and their means to eat. That's not right in my opinion.

The mandate to mask-up for everybody was a powerful move and smart just because you have the vaccine it doesn't mean to much of nothing except you can carry it, and pass it, and you can still get it so, mask up for the rest of the world and be a nice human being you'll be blessed for it.

I'm so excited about having things to do when I get out of this hospital and more excited to physically be able to volunteer here and publish this book. Just a couple of items on the to-do list. Here's a big one ..., plan for my wedding next year! I'm so excited that I can barely wait! When the heavens drop an angel into your arms and you don't wrap your arms securely around him or she..., you don't deserve one day with them. So, she is securely wrapped and swaddled with every ounce of everything I can give her right now. Gotta start the search for "Thatguy Rcurtis Show" (my talk show I've had since March 17,2020 Covid chaos beginnings). I've got to prepare for motivational speaking so many things in God's time though so, it will all be complete.

You know how good it feels to smile and tell someone to have a fantastic day and mean it like for real mean it? It is a very satisfying feeling, and it really makes your day that more enjoyable and stress free. Try it sometimes and notice your whole disposition and attitude change even on a stormy day it will feel like 80-degree weather! That is so dope! Yeah, great attitude. In my business of helping people buy transportation for their family's needs attitude is my number one success module if I don't start with a good attitude my day is ruined by someone coming in with a horrible nasty attitude and all because of me and my lack of preparing for my day. "If you stay ready, you don't have to get ready" and that is why that person that comes in with the bad attitude loses because I was not prepared to give them the service, they needed to get up out of their funk for the day. My fault, my 'L' I hate losing! 'Winners always make it happen; losers always make excuses." When the economy went bad, I did not blame the economy I blamed me!

When they say the car business is bad all over, I do not allow that to reach my Inner cortex of my cerebral NOPE! I blame me for not contacting enough prospects and prior clients. I'm a Winner! I'm a leader! I don't make excuses, I get my motivation from all objections, and I figure out how to overcome them! That is why I'm successful in life! Amen.

God takes care of me at all costs because I take care of his children at all costs. So, if you see me and you truly need something…., I got you!

Out of sight out of mind this is the concept I decided to use with my recovery. I figured people had other things to do instead of keeping track of my every move and me having to report every step. What is that? I just want to get better and get out and get straight to my business. I'm so excited about my responsibilities and my new agenda! I think I'm being a little redundant now but, I am excited!

When a giant gets rest, he develops a plethora of energy he can now use to start his task. That giant 22 days (about 3 weeks) in this hospital has gotten me rested and ready for action, mentally, physically, spiritually, and emotionally. Let's go!

I WILL SLEEP WHEN I AM DEAD.

I believe I heard that from a preacher before and it stuck with me ever since I heard it. I don't recall who the preacher was that said it, but it resonated with them as it does to this day. To me it made sense because, I don't need that much sleep, we just require a little rest to make it. 6,8 or more hours of rest is (to me) a little much. After taking a little 15-minute nap I'm good and as long as I get about 4 hours rest, I'm Gucci as the young people say. Ready to go!

Let me explain to you what I mean by GIANTs. Ok, to me there are a select few who have been chosen to be leaders and guide the rest of many who are lost and confused and need help to maintain or be redirected to their path. This is one of the GIANTs responsibilities, listening and leading by example is the absolute most important one of all!

Barry White (may he RIP) said it best with his hit song, "Practice what you preach" obviously he had a different connotation, tone and agenda behind his lyrics or so he thought..., the message was still conveyed. When you are constantly attempting to do your part in this thing as one of the chosen few, it gets exhausting, and you are so focused that you neglect your own self so, since your "soul partner" is unable to get you to slow down, sometimes your father in Heaven, your higher power, your supreme being, your go-to has to lay you down to get you prepared for the next phase, the level, the mission, hence even a GIANT needs rest.

A pilot can't fly an aircraft while exhausted or that pilot will be putting all of the passengers at risk.

A surgeon definitely can't operate on someone while needing to get a little shut-eye or that surgeon will more than likely end a life instead of saving it.

A preacher cannot deliver a sermon that is going to be effective without experiencing a proper slumber.

And a messenger cannot deliver a solid message and travel the world spreading the "good news" without much needed rest.

Can you perform your necessary duties efficiently if you're sleepy, tired, hungover, not well rested, angry from tossing and turning? I'll help you right here because we don't have time for you to ponder the obvious.... NO, you can't!

And without adequate rest nor can the GIANTs amongst us who have a tremendous job to complete.

We are only human.

CHAPTER TEN

We made it! Day 25 and I'm going home! Yeh! You know I never had any doubt that I'd be getting out of the hospital just overly anxious as to when I would be getting out. Well, my oxygen needs are obviously to the Doctor's satisfaction so, today is the day! It's funny because the same doctor came into my room yesterday and said, "Are you ready to go home?" I said yes, I am. And he responds with "ok maybe tomorrow." What a jerk I thought then I got over it. I don't know what the percentage of patients with Covid are in an induced coma on a breathing machine but, that seems to be the "go to" for the treatment. I thank God, he brought me through this! It was not an easy ordeal and at times just a little too much for your boy to take but, we got through it and I'm telling you not on my worst enemy do I wish this.

I had physical therapy today and well you know I'm going to push it as far as I can for some extraordinary results, and I got just that. Colleen was extremely impressed with my progress especially after laying down for the beginning of my stay to now walking back and forth in my room. Those push-ups and that active lifestyle of mine helped. Man, but did I lose some weight…, I lost about twenty pounds at least, I'm straight up and down sideways and I have "noassatall" legs are all skinny to me I look funny, and I laugh every time I look at myself in the mirror because I know this is also temporary your boy is getting back on the saddle and getting his physique back. One thing I do love is my stomach is flat! Now, it has been thirty plus years since my stomach has been flat so, you know I'll be adding some sit-ups to the regimen to keep that as flat as I can;

six packs I don't care about that. I do want to be able to see my shoe size though…. Lol!

I'm so excited about getting out of this hospital tomorrow I decided to go to sleep early. I still was waking up throughout the night. I laid down after Sunday Night Football then I woke up at eleven, two am, four fifteen or so and then I finally said forget it and got up at six something. It was cool. I needed to proofread the book, check on some emails, do some breathing exercises and some more stuff. So, it worked out fine. I always would try to text my kids my progress every morning so they would not worry as much, keep my moms posted as well. Could not do too much talking that would take my breath away. That was a bit challenging for me but guess what I did what I needed to do.

It's about ten thirty and in comes Colleen, my physical therapist; I thought she was off for the weekend nope; she is here for a final analysis of my condition. "Ok, you ready? " she says? Yep, give me a few seconds to regulate my breathing. Here's the thing whenever I said that I was hurting myself because I was telling the rest of my body that it was time for me to have a violent episode of coughing as soon as I said that the coughing began. Crazy, huh? Not really because our mouths tell our brains what to relay to the rest of our body. That's real talk you guys. If you tell your body that it is about to be sick it will get sick. Our mouths are powerful, and our brains can play so many tricks on us since it is constantly being programmed and re-programed.

Before this Covid fiasco I would get sick once every three years and even then, it is just a little cold or something; no joke. I was in church back in nineteen ninety-six or so and we had a pastor visiting from down south. It was Alabama or Oklahoma or something like that. I remember him saying something like, "I don't get sick, because I don't speak things like that into existence for myself." That was it for me, no more getting sick. If I don't speak then it will not happen. Believe or not ever since that day that I took on that attitude I did not get sick anymore.

Now this Covid is another animal.

I'm not claiming to be sick of this either, it was just time for me to get some rest because you know even a giant needs rest and then get well stronger than I was before and get to the work that I have been instructed to do. Some of you guy's and gal's might not understand what I mean, so as to not keep you in the dark while you are trying to enjoy my book, I will say it again in plain language. God sat me down so that he could prepare me physically, mentally, and spiritually for my journey ahead for his kingdom. There, I hope that made it more clear for you.

Man, I cannot wait to get started!

Books, music, motivational speaking, advocate for Covid patients and so much more!

First, get the heck out this hospital! I called Natasha and told her it would be about ten thirty or eleven but, then I had to tell her it is going to be later because the company with the oxygen machine is in Seattle and the delivery person lives in Kent but had to pick up the machine from Seattle and she is stuck in traffic, but she will be here after that. Really??? Plus, the Doctor is playing a game. He has not been in my room at all this morning so, I hit the nurses button and she comes to the door. "May I help you, your button is on?" "Yes, any idea when the doctor will be in here to release me?" Before she could begin her response, he's right there behind her. After he gave me his story, he then had the audacity to say, "don't be surprised if you don't go home today because I can't get the breathing machine." I stopped him right in his words and said, "don't put a "but" or an "if" in the sentence because it negates things" he kept on so then I said, "I'm getting out of this hospital today by hook or crook" yesterday you'd played a game talking you want to go home and then you gon' say maybe tomorrow, we rebuking Satan with the blood of Jesus that machine will be here and I will be going home today" as he's walking out he's like "ok." Don't get me wrong I was not loud or mean just direct I was even smiling and whispering with these lungs. So, it was cool. About three or so in the afternoon I got out.

Have you ever just been so in awe of fresh air that you want it all over your face and body and inside your soul? It just felt so good to be out in the elements. Y'all just don't know man, I wanted to kiss the ground but, it would have been hard for me to get back up with my now skinny behind... Lol I'm out! God did what he said he was going to do; take care of me! The first thing I did was obvious. I hugged my baby as much as I could with the oxygen machine on my lap along with the rest of my belongings while in a wheelchair. The second thing I did was get in the car and open the window, the moonroof and just take in the breeze and sun rays. I could not stop smiling and thanking God and saying hallelujah! I was so happy and free, and it felt good!

Now, the drive home was a little different for whatever reason we missed each other so much we did not know what to say or talk about nevertheless it was a great ride to the house. Everything looked so different and new to me. It has been thirty plus day's since I've driven a car or walked outside or just sat outside in the back yard or on the front porch. In time my friend, in time. Ok, here we are. I'm greeted with a distant hello because nobody knows if I'm still contagious. I know because I inquired, I thought it was funny then Natasha says, "you can give him a hug" so here we go... the love is the part. If not for the love the willingness to fight would not have been there.

Now, it is time to get out of the car and walk up stairs into the house. When I tell you guys that was no way near easy, I mean that just that. I was out of breath when I got to the top of the stairs. Colleen said something about that today during P/T. She said we are going to step up on this ledge type of thing it was about maybe a foot and a half off the ground, and she was telling me how one of her patience did not hold on to the handle and had a little spill and it was because her muscles had forgotten how to step up. So, I heard her and yes, I held on to the handle and what was crazy is I felt my leg and calf muscles trying to adjust while I was lifting my leg to climb up and when I landed, I felt it in my leg like it damn near gave out. Crazy! Me,

Mr. got my momma's butt and thighs! Not no more.... It's gone. Whatever, I'll be back better than I ever was, trust me on that!

I make it to the couch and I feel nasty because I have not been able to take a shower the whole time, got a little I forget what they called it but some acronym they used, it meant they use some wipes and gave you what is commonly known as a "hoe bath" a wipe up and that it is not at all cool in my book so, the first thing I want to do is get in the Jacuzzi tub and soak because I don't have the energy to stand in the shower yet. Mind you that's fifteen stairs to conquer.... Whew! I think I'll eat first. I told Natasha what I wanted for dinner when I got out and she granted my request. Her bomb chicken and some home-made French fries! I could not taste anything! I must have been working with memory because I maxed that food and had seconds! It is so good to be home Y'all I'm telling you! I don't normally watch tv, I will watch some football though and that is what I did although I really wanted to get in that tub. Those fifteen flights of stairs were very intimidating, and it forced me to wait until I just could not take it any more.

About a half an hour after the game I decided to brave those stairs. I grabbed the rail I started up. I did not stop until I got to the top then it was a violent cough, regulate your breathing time. Now, this one right here hurts and it made me hot and frustrated. It took about three minutes or so for me to calm down and remember there is nothing no one can do for you while you are going through these episodes. It is all on you so, I call on the holy ghost for a little help. Ain't nobody playing! A simple "help me holy ghost" does wonder's! You still gotta go through it though it just relieves your mind while you settle down. The water is ready, and I am not, because now I got to walk another fifteen feet to the tub.

I do it and have another fit in the tub for about maybe three minutes or so then I calm down and turn on the jets. Ahh, the water is hot, and the jets are massaging my body oh yeah, I forgot to mention that since I was not completely cleaned in the hospital and toward the end I was mostly sitting in a chair until I decided to lay in the bed well not only did your boy get hemorrhoids from straining and being backed up, but he also had like bed sores in the crack of his (no) ass! You're serious right now??!!?? Yes, I am and let me talk about that type of pain. I'm fifty-six years old and I don't believe I've ever experienced pain like that before, especially around that region of my body. It burns, burns, burns, and doesn't stop because it is raw, I'm only glad that I did not get some type of infection from that. Anyway, so I'm enjoying my bath and trying to adjust so that I can work through this booty pain. I'm out though and in good health just got to continue to stay encouraged knowing God got me. Every now and again I'm in my head it would try to mess with me and have me thinking about folk who make it home from the hospital then pass away from something they did or something the hospital missed. You know how we are as human beings. We're always in our own heads making things more than what they really are.

I'm in the tub an hour or so Natasha says, "are you ready?" "Nope let me chill for a little bit longer babe" my ass is killing me!

Man, I'm telling you I do not wish this on my very first enemy that I acquired in pre-school! I am so serious! This whole thing is a testimony and I'm going to tell it like it, T-I-is – the late great Bernie Mac.

I get out of the tub, I'm standing, and my caregiver is drying me off. I'm trying not to cough you guys. It isn't easy plus it is good for me to cough because it is opening different passages to my lungs. When you are coughing as violently as I was, you care but you don't care because it hurts to cough like that! Anyway, now I'm lying on the bed getting treated for ass bed sores. You know you have a real woman when she doesn't even think twice about how gross this is going to be she goes right in to aid you in getting better doing whatever she can. This is so dope, I'm so loved and I love her so much too!

No, I'm not going to get all mushy on Y'all let's get back into the situation. Coughing episodes when I get to the bed and what makes it uncomfortable and painful is the fact that my lungs are attempting to open different passageways; however, the ones that are not open yet are so closed that when I cough those joker's are painful right in my neck close to my lungs! So, that's why hate coughing. Walking to the bathroom is no picnic either it is weird though because even though I feel like I have enough energy and strength to do it is still like climbing those fifteen stairs to me at first now, I got it down. I'm day five at home and I'm only on two percent oxygen and I'm sitting up going to the bathroom and showering but I still got quite a way to go. Yesterday I decided to tackle the fifteen stairs and chill on the couch and eat dinner at the table. It was cool no violent coughing there was a little coughing because like I told you guys I have to cough it means I'm healing. That felt good! It really felt like I accomplished something! Oh yeah!

I figured something out yesterday too. There is this lung exercise apparatus that is used to help open your lungs (I forget the name of it) . I could look it up but I'm not. Whatever! That's not important right now, what is important is what I figured out yesterday. I figured out that it is not the exhaling that's important, it is the inhaling that will expand my lungs and help me off this oxygen machine a lot sooner than normal. Now I'm inhaling and holding my breath about ten to fifteen times an hour, and it is helping with controlling my coughs and it is helping me with getting out of my head! I was so excited when I figured that out and saw positive results from it, I did not know what to do!

That's when I said I'm going downstairs and eating dinner and chilling and that's what I did. Took my time about going back up though. The funny thing is when I decided to walk back up man, my legs did that thing again and I was like whoa did not feel like I was going to fall or anything it just felt like my legs were bending in slow motion. Weird! It's going to take some time to get in motion; time is what I have plenty of now, can't work and that's killing me so, I'm up every morning at five am working like I have a job and I do have a job even though it's not selling cars right now it is getting my business erected and getting publishing for this book and submitting songs and researching different avenues for venues and speaking engagements and checking on my 501c3 nonprofit progress and a host of other things see I don't know how to just lay here and take it that's not how I was designed so, let's get to work young man! I really thought my book was completed in the hospital I guess I should have considered the fact I was writing on my iPhone notepad and that I did not have that many pages written found that out today when amazon said it had to be a minimum of seventy-five pages and I was at twelve or fifteen Lmao!

Oh, well all I could do is continue right, right so that is now what I am doing.

I'm giving you guys a play-by-play on my recovery. Well, my (no) ass is healing and my hemorrhoids are shrinking and I'm able to get into the shower and let the water run on my face, I'm going back down the fifteen stairs for some uno tonight can't freakin have a glass of wine or beer because of my medicine I guess plus my care provider is not having it. Oh well it has been damn near close to thirty days since I had a drink or a tree. Guess I'm not hooked on either one; no withdrawals... Lol!

Blood thinner, steroids, stool softener all the medication I'm on right now. I can remember wondering as a kid how my Nana (RIH) could take all of these pills at once. Now I'm doing it, not to mention my caregiver got me some vitamins, and magnesium, I forget what else it is working though because I am making great progress and feeling good!

Can you imagine going from needing one hundred percent oxygen to two percent oxygen it is an amazing feeling that can't be described kind of like an old girlfriend years ago who asked me how it felt when a man released, I knew there was not a way to explain it in words so, I put my hand over her mouth and nose and held it until she had to gasp for air and said like that. She said, "oh." You think she got it though? Sorry about that it was little much I guess; it just came to me as I was explaining to you guys how it felt to breathe again.

Forgive me. I have been sitting on this bed since five am this morning. It is now three twenty-four in the afternoon. Natasha is off work and I believe cooking dinner or on the phone talking to one of her friends. I'm determined to get this book published not now but, right now Amazon! I'm learning a lot about myself while I'm keeping you all abreast of my progress. I'm for the most a patient fella... not! Ok, I'm focus driven, not a slouch, know how to keep a flow of income coming in, not easily let down, don't really take no for an answer when it comes to what I want to accomplish, professional, goal driven, talented, cool, open, loving, forgiving, spiritual, kind, zero tolerance for bullshit type of guy and strong.

Just a few things that I've learned and confirmed.

I had a bowel movement today!!! I Have not had a real one on my own for about three and a half weeks. I was not in any health danger though because if you recall earlier, I had said I had not eaten anything four days before the hospital and four days' while in the hospital so, I had no waste to get rid of since I've been home though, home cooked meals every day! Breakfast, lunch, and dinner! Man, I'll tell you what, "it's good to be the king especially when you have a tremendous queen by your side!"

Yesterday I took a walk on the wild side; no oxygen and went to the mall. It was a little much the walking oh, I did use the portable oxygen for that did not want to take a chance of "needing and not having." I walked about a total of two hundred to two-hundred fifty feet to and from the car and had a little coughing episode then it was under control in a matter of seconds. See you guys I was determined to buy Natasha her engagement ring as soon as I got out of the hospital which obviously was impossible so, first chance I felt like let's do it, that's what we did. Found the one she wanted online, and they had it in the store! So, we went to the mall. She was totally against it all the way to the mall once my mind was set though there is nothing anyone can say or do to change it.

We took all the necessary precautions like the portable oxygen, and she dropped me off at the door, we had our masks on and we took it super slow. I did not have to wait in line, just asked for the lady we spoke to on the phone, and the transaction took place. I told her, " I've been in the car business for over thirty -five years and I don't pay retail for anything, I usually negotiate with my current condition I'm not in the frame of health to do that right now so, congratulations on your sale" she said, "oh, no I'm going to get you some discounts that way when I need a car you can return the favor" now that right there what she did and how she presented was pure "great customer service" and she is now my jeweler. It doesn't take much to satisfy a real customer who is just looking for someone to spend money with. Kill them with "country kindness" , listen and deliver what you said you were going to do. Too easy – J Cole.

I got down on one knee without even thinking twice and put the ring on Natasha's finger then slowly got back up...Lol.

Her smile was so precious, and it made me satisfied. Ok, back in the car back to the house where there was a "home-made" apple pie cooling down in the window and "home-made chicken noodle soup to be eaten" oh yeah, and the rest of the Sea Hawks game to watch! The Tennessee Titans come back twenty-four nine to win in overtime thirty-three thirty! Win, lose or draw they are still my team man, they be, pissing me off though I just want them to have that "fight until the game is over and don't let up" attitude. It's all good.

CHAPTER ELEVEN

That boy Lamar Jackson is a freakin phenom though and my guy Patrick Mahomes is nice as well. I was not rooting for either of the teams. I just like watching those quarterbacks play. Well now it is time to tackle those fifteen stairs. I get to the top and have a little cough then it calms down. It takes a little more time because I think it's reflecting on the mall walk which I will not be doing again anytime soon. I slept half the night with the oxygen and half without it. I'm weaning off this thing although I know it is not, it feels like an enabler to me so, I'm figuring out ways of breathing exercises and techniques to help open other passageways to my lungs and taking it slow still not doing too much on purpose. It seems to be working out for me too. No oxygen this morning woke up peed, and thought I had to take a dump, nope..., just air. Got right to work. Did my flier for "Thatguy Rcurtis Show" did some social media promoting, handled some medical financial business, ate breakfast, took my meds, started writing in the book.

You know why I produced the title I did for this book? Well, first because Covid does physically hurt. Mostly though because of everything that I experienced while in the hospital. Hearing about the other patients that did not have a great support crew or prayer warriors and they are all alone because they did not have a belief system so therefore got in their heads and never came out now, they are in an induced coma fighting for their lives with a hose down their throat.

Then there was the silence oh, the silence which allowed for deep thinking and the wondering what I can do to help instead of talking about helping, then there were the children…. That did it right there, that's the biggest hurt of them all because it just doesn't make any sense that we gave up on them so, they gave up on themselves and that's not right so, a lot of my hurt with Covid had a lot to do with that and man and woman's selfishness when it comes to masking up. Now, I know I'm not supposed to focus on things that I can't control; however, this is something that I can help advocate for and change one or two minds on the subject matter. There are so many different scenarios in our world that need to be addressed and they will be accordingly. That is where the name came from all of that incorporated with the physical, mental, and spiritual hurt of Covid. My personal experience will aid in helping someone else make it through the dreadful Covid experience like I did. Who knows? All I know is I'm going to do my part and put it out here just as raw as I went through it that way you can't get it misconstrued or confused.

If you can imagine this and visualize at the same time, I was just sitting with my hand under my chin trying to think where to go from there and I chuckled because so far, it has just been flowing, I must be in my head again. "Satan, I rebuke you with the blood of Jesus!" I often say that aloud to get him off me and it works until he decides to try again then I just say it again. Did you know every time I say it, he must flee?

Facts. He can come back as many times as he wants though. Be strong, be diligent, be faithful, know and believe that "no weapons formed against you shall prosper" and you too will make it out of a Covid type situation better than you went into it. Trust me, I'm a witness and a survivor.

Sent out invites for the engagement party last night and this morning we got a lot of congratulations and I talked to her dad for the first time (he lives in Texas) he was incredibly happy for us. He was telling her how proud he was of her for stepping up to the plate and doing what most women would have not had the strength emotionally, mentally, or physically to do. I told her the same thing because I too realized what she did was remarkable, and I so appreciated that she had that in her. Anyway, he continued, he was happy for us then he asked to speak to his daughter so, off speaker and she went into her office. I had an after-thought of the traditional "sir may I have your blessings and your permission for your daughters' hand in marriage" then I said Nawl, that's corny plus he was cool with the news. Sometimes you can do too much, and this was a time that less was more. Along with this book I also will be releasing three songs, "Permanent Situation", " If you want it" and "Christmas Melodies" all written, produced, composed and sung by me. Along with the song's I will also have videos for them all. So, now you see my work is cut-out for me. Not that it matters I'm sure some of you are thinking, "at your age"? The thing is with the way social media and the world is today, age doesn't matter its presentation and content along with uniqueness.

So, yes at my age! Now, it is time to get to work and share these gifts of mine with you all! I'm not at all interested in being buried with any of them. I remember when I used to say I don't know who to talk to or contact to get my stuff out there, now it is nothing to put a song out on the market. It is all about the follow through and the marketing strategy which I will be needing help with. Although, when I was promoting, it was me in marketing and we did damned good in the money department, but that's history and this is now so let's go!

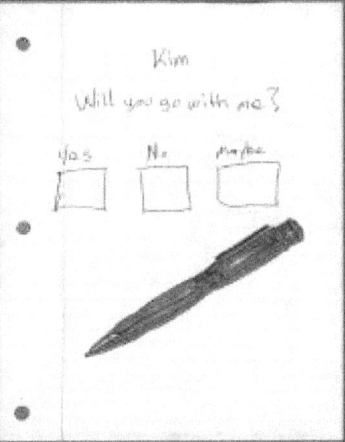

CHAPTER TWELVE

Covid will make you think about your life in a glimpse, and you will make changes or not. I chose to make changes. I'm sitting up here and can't really do too much of anything so, why just be a bump on a log when I can be productive in other ways such as, this book, my songs, my show. I've done more resting (for myself) than I did when I was healthy and strong! It's amazing the little things that you can do after going through what I did just seem to stick out in your mind. For example, brushing my teeth while standing in the bathroom, standing in the shower, and having strength to hold my head down while the water runs down my neck, lifting me out of bed to go to the bathroom to pee and not losing my breath. The little things, the simple pleasure in life that we typically don't think twice about, we just feel like that's supposed to happen automatically, that's normal. Well, you guys I got news for you, it is not supposed to just happen, and it is not normal, it is taken for granted though by all of us.

Look at it this way, some people don't pray because they say, "I don't know what to pray about." How about just saying thank you for your life? Since you know tomorrow is not promised; start there and then it will just start flowing. Prayer is just like a conversation you have with anybody. It just intimidates a lot of us because it is God and we know we've done something, so we are scared to talk to God; the one who said, "I forgive you" and things of that nature. God is our parent, and you are not afraid to talk to them regardless of what you did last night. Consider the fact that he already knew what you were going to do before you had the thought in your mind about doing it so, ask for forgiveness, forgive yourself and build a beautiful relationship with your dad; "he can, get you right!"

You know what? If I had my life to do all over again, I would not change anything because there is no telling where I would be in my life at this minute if I changed one millisecond of it. And where I am right now mentally and spiritually, I love it, Covid recovery and all! I've never in my life felt so focused and driven to do so many things and get them all done, ever! I feel so free and light like there is nothing I can't do! I feel like I'm getting stronger and stronger every day, and I will be stronger than I was before, mentally, and physically. I'll tell you one thing for sure; I am now as happy on the outside as I am on the inside and that my friends "is" the most!

I'm sitting here with no oxygen machine; I'm breathing on my own! No complications, no shortness of breath, just breathing normal, this is awesome! I am eight days out of the hospital and making this rapid progress. "Like I say" in the words of Big C (RIH), God don't half -step ladies and gents he is all or nothing!

He will make your enemies your footstools, whoa! That's some power right there!

That's love right there!

That's a bomb relationship right there! Enemies, your footstools... wow!

Anyway, I am eight days in and I'm feeling great!

My (noassatall) bed sores are healing... Lol!

And it's just beautiful to look out my window and see the clouds, rain, and the concrete.

The day before my born day.

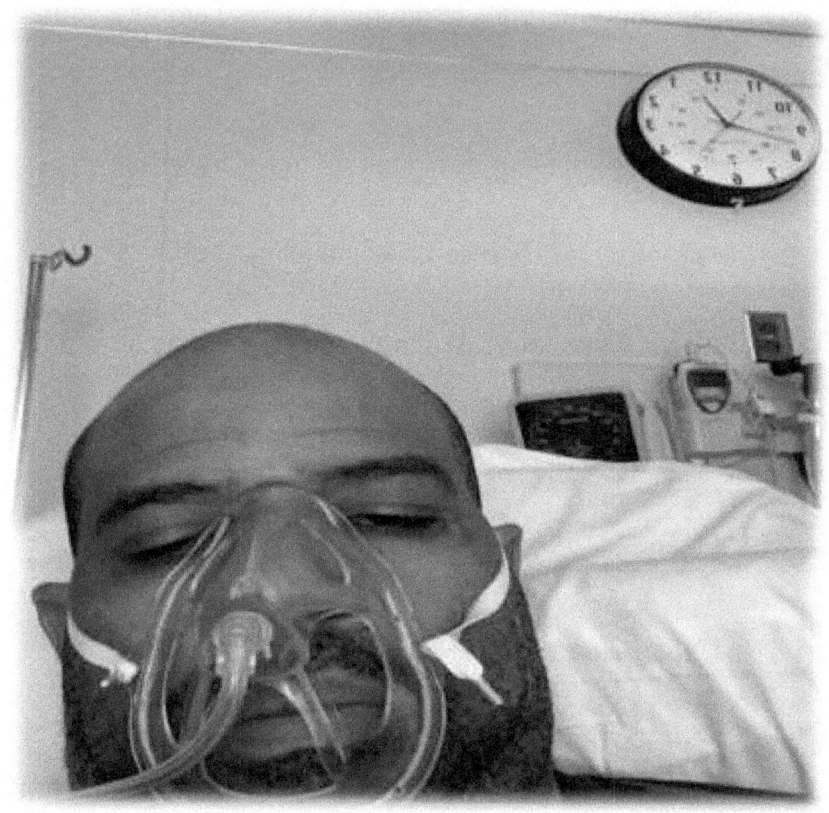

Me in ICU with the high flow oxygen I'm at one hundred percent oxygen, I'm not breathing at all on my own.

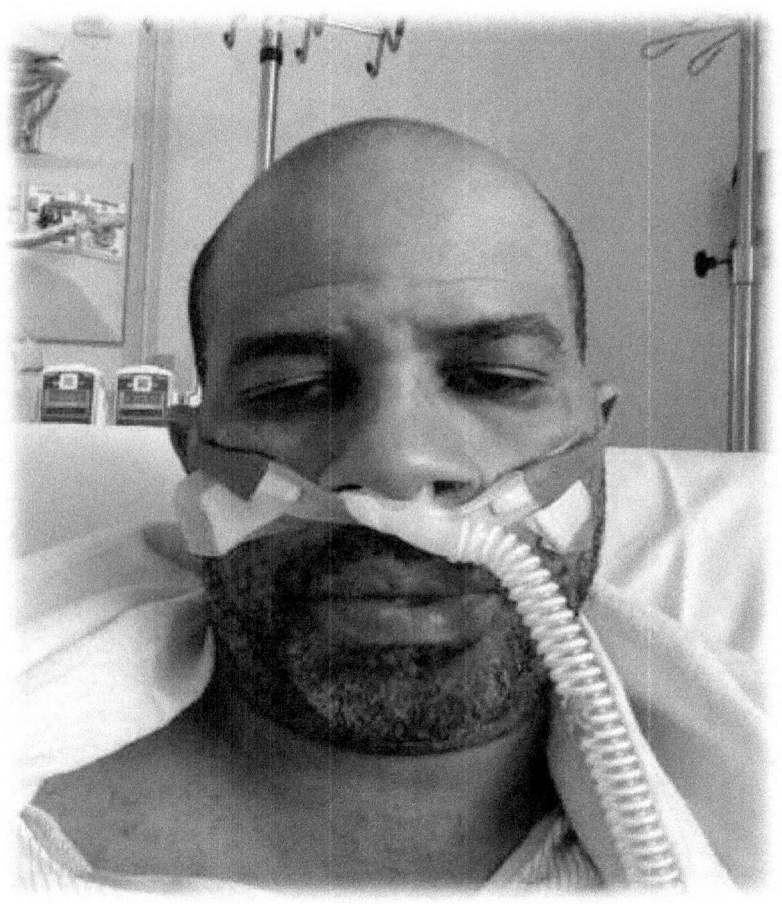

This is me when I found out I was going home in one to two days!

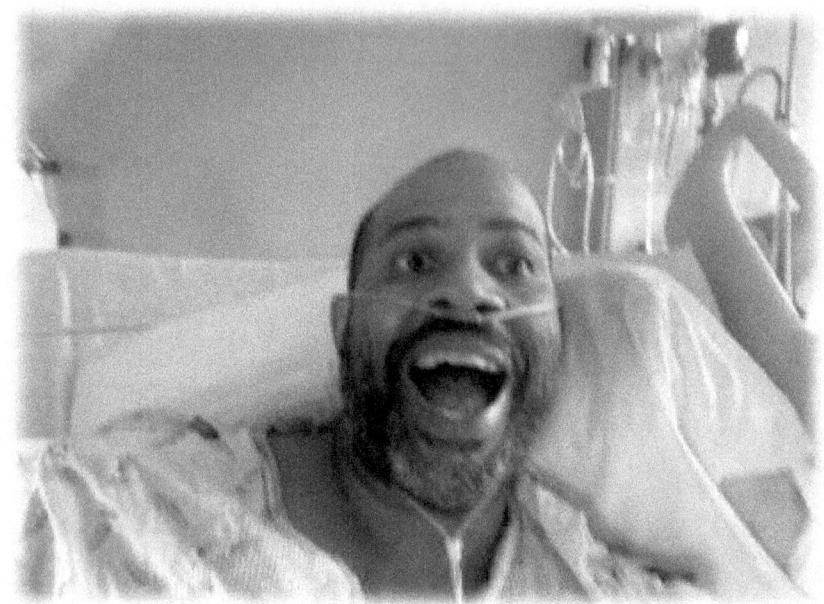

First day of out of ICU doing a breathing treatment reppin'
Sea Hawks!

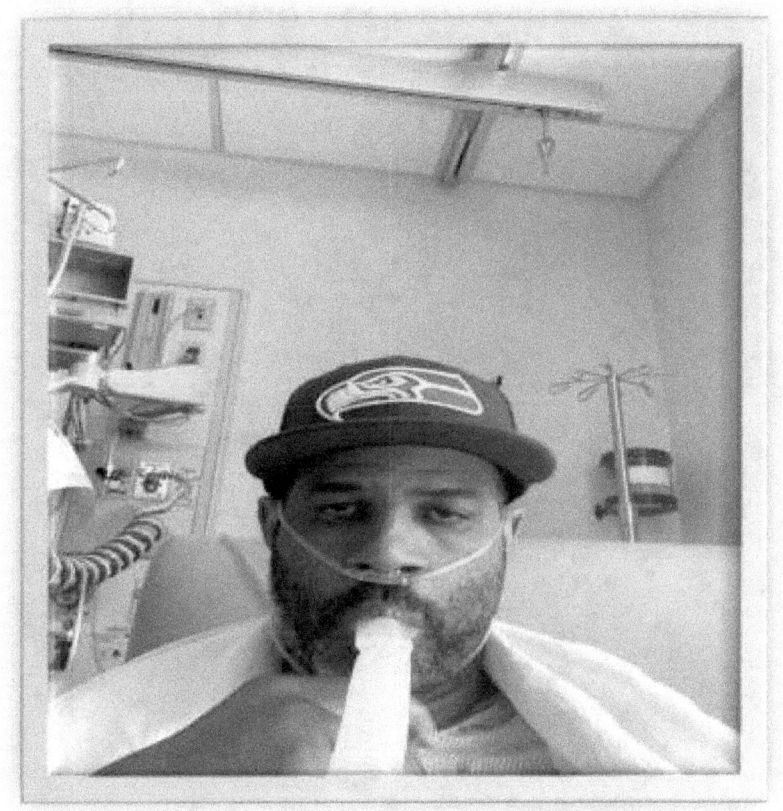

The home / portable oxygen set-up.

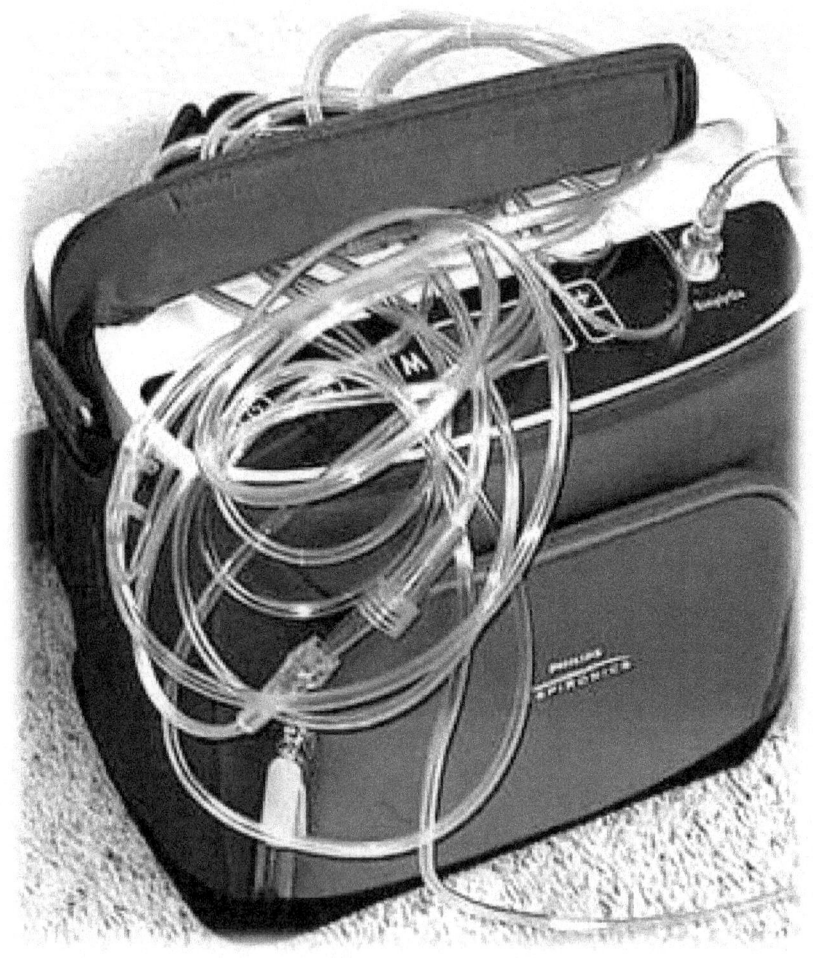

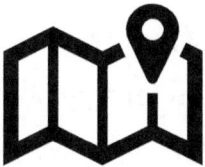

CHAPTER THIRTEEN

When you are down that never means you are out it just means that you are rejuvenating for the rest of the race. I have not stopped working since I got out of the hospital, and it feels damned good! I refuse to be enabled due to a minor / major set-back I now know how those who are physically handicapped refuse to be called handicap and don't like to live handicapped. Hat's off to them! Your circumstance should not dictate the rest of your life and your accomplishments never! It's what you do with them that matters if you are the type to just lay there and take it, complain about everything not going right and you don't know how to look at the bright side of things.... You should seek psychological help from a professional. I'm profoundly serious because there is no reason for a person to just be negative all the time. You are breathing on your own, so you have an opportunity to create some change in your life that's reason enough to half-way smile anyway. Don't wait, do it now!

So, like I said I have not stopped working since I got out of the hospital, not physically administrative work for "Thatguy Rcurtis Show" and on my music releases, on video storyboards I mean non-stop sometimes fifteen hours a day! This is what I'm supposed to be doing working my brain and growing more knowledgeable, more focused, more- hungry and not waiting for someone to come along to "save me."

I am very well capable of holding my own trust and believe. This is when I change the energy circle if it is not beneficial, cancel credit cards that don't benefit me, change telephone companies if the customer service "sucks" Verizon (my opinion based on my personal experience), and move on to the next chapter without looking back. Afterall, you have already been there so why look back? Nothing there, just what you wanted to leave behind. Let's get more motivated to leave well enough alone and move forward to the next opportunity, the blessing to follow, the getting better while in a better situation! Don't stop hustling, grinding with the tenacity of a winner. Write stuff down you would like to accomplish TODAY not the rest of the week. How do you clean your house? I'm sure if you are efficient, it is room -to -room making sure it's completed before you make your way to the next room. If not, then you are all confused within your own head, and you need to get that dead weight off you so that what's inside you can come out and finish the work you are supposed to be doing!

It's not rocket science, it is basic common sense: you can't make it on your own. You need divine coverage and divine guidance from the creator of all men, women, children, animals, and the skies.

If you are attempting to do this walk on your own, you may make it. It's going to be a tough one for you though when all you had to do was open your mouth and ask for your path..., no one else's just your own then it is a whole lot easier and it's enjoyable at times too!

"When God says he got you, he got you" and not in a haphazard like way either.

Day 12 no oxygen, walking on my own without any assistance, killing these fifteen stairs, I even drove a couple of days ago (with accompaniment) the coughs are a little more frequent due to my lungs expeditiously opening; however, my physical strength is not back yet and honestly, I don't expect it back until next month. At least that's when I plan to return to work to start getting my money again…. My pay was cut eighty percent last month; then God!

He gave me all my money back with some interest. Ya dig!

He doesn't half-step and he can't lie so he said he got me and that he does in every aspect of the term and definition! Awesome! Spoke to my mom briefly last night about 9 pm or so. Tell me something, does your mom feel like she must constantly remind you she is your mom? I'm simply curious because it never fails sometime during a visit or a call that natural born fact will spew out of her mouth for any random reason don't get me wrong it is not like she just be coming out her all willy-nilly with gibberish no, that's not it all she has Napoleon complex and thinks she must input fear in my heart or something. It's funny to me because I've known you now for fifty-six years and still don't know you because we don't know how to communicate with each other and that's fine and at the same time not ok. I just learned how to deal with the fact that I may never know who my mom is I still love you and will do anything for you and that's out of the respect that I have for you, not as my mom but as my mom and a strong black queen who made it out here on her own and needed no one by her side just God and I admire that. I will always honor your strength and your tenacity along with your love for others.

The issue is listening and responding instead of cutting off and reacting. And I think when it comes to our relationship, we are both guilty of it.

I hope she reads my book otherwise that was random; needed to be released though.

I get a lot of people asking about the vaccine now that I've had Covid. I think that's interesting because they feel like I should fear covid enough to RUN TO THE VACCINE for safety. I don't know how you guys operate. I don't operate that way. I was not designed with fear in my body so therefore I don't put it in my body. I think that the vaccine should be like politics not to be discussed except privately amongst your circle of friends. There are too many people that are for the vaccine and still refuse to wear a mask and that to me is SUPER funny. How are you going to dictate to people on how to save the world and you are breathing your whole soul on them at the grocery store and the restaurant! Double standards and selfishness and I'm supposed to take advice for my health from you? Get outta here! I wanted to cuss so bad right there I just decided that it was not necessary. I think I'm getting my point across quite clearly. So, the next time you decide (if you are one of those selfish souls) to walk up to me and tell me I don't have to wear a mask if I'm vaccinated, or you stand less than six feet away from me with no mask. Save your breath and watch your step because I'm a weirdo and I'll say something sarcastic and prophetic that will make you want to get violent don't do that though because we both have way too much to lose and neither one of us is worth it. So just mind your business and your step's and with your thoughts be safe.

That had to come out too.

I'm picking up weight again, my stomach is not as flat as it was when I came home from the hospital, I can still see my shoe size though... Lol! My legs are still Hella skinny, and my chest is flat. It's all good though this is just motivation to utilize my gym equipment and be back better than I was before!

You will see if you know me and if not, you'll see because it will be broadcasted on "Thatguy Rcurtis Show" (Shameless plug) wait a minute I'm not ashamed.... Lol!

Remember how I said earlier you must have a great support team to make it through the whole covid fiasco? Well, it is true. Since I got home, I've been taken care of to the fullest, not coddled or spoiled, just gotten all my needs taken care of; medication, vitamins, four meals a day like that. My show has been handled by my assistant Lil Homie and she has been doing a stellar job. I mean I would have never guessed that she would be a natural.... Amazing! She just wants to be behind the scenes though and I can respect that; however, she might have to piggyback a showoff of "Thatguy Rcurtis Show" and would not be against in the least bit! That's how you grow by sprouting out and spreading seeds.

Also, that's how you get your blessings to keep on coming.

God don't halfway do nothing!

If you take a picture of this QR code, you can upload my app and watch "Thatguy Rcurtis Show " past and present.

I just thought I would share and what better way to get to new viewers and listeners than by allowing access in my book?

ABC – always be closing!

DBS – don't be stupid (Lol)

YOGOC – You only get one chance

TAOAO – Take advantage of all opportunities

Ok, I'm done with that, cool acronyms though if I may say so myself.

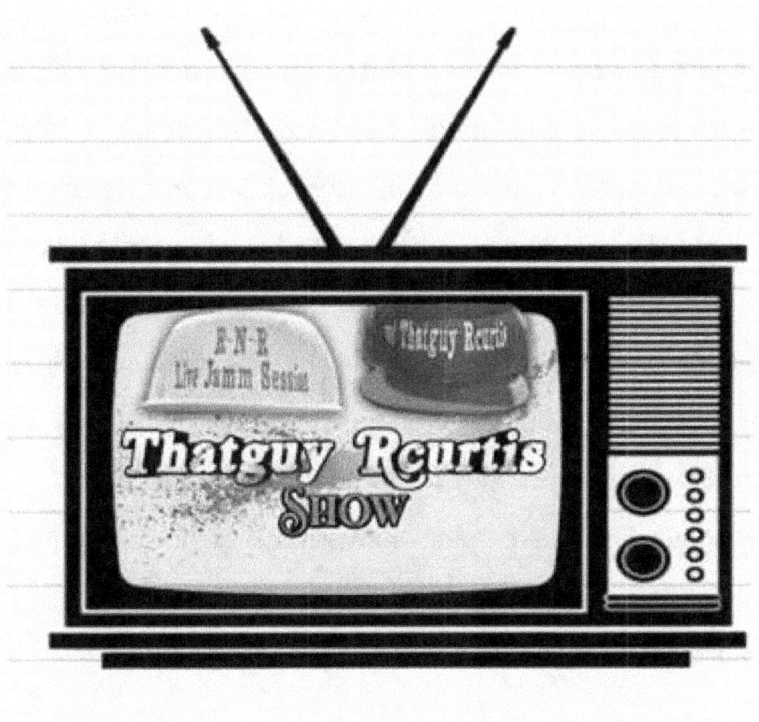

If I said to you that my life is the way it is supposed to be right now, and I'm totally pleased with it. What would you think, would you just assume that my finances are close to perfect, or would you think that my soul is so filled that I am overjoyed? Well, let me help you out, it is the latter. I wake up every morning now about 4:30 am and have such an enjoyable conversation with God that my soul is filled, and I am overjoyed which makes it easy to have a better day. And my conversations with him are different now; they are more like check ins, confirmations, and directions. It's so much easier to pray now, I love it! Since I've been out of the hospital and been recovering from Covid I have gotten the news of about five or six people dying from this evil disease! I don't know what to say except for; "make sure your relationship is right with the creator" seriously, you don't want to leave this earth not knowing where you are going and with this Covid spreading and now they have another one that has been created and released like a new movie... mmm, mmm, mmm.

Why make something like this and then announce it and just sit back and watch your creation destroy and take lives? It's EVIL there is no other reason to wreak havoc on the world like this, no reason! So, now you see what I mean about making sure your relationship is good with the creator? I hope so, because at the end of the day if you are reading my book then you can't say you did not know because the information has been presented to you.

I loss a Patna' to Covid two days ago I didn't even know, Slim used to check on me all the time and the same day he dies from Covid was the day that I was thinking man, Slim hasn't called me and I was thinking about checking in with him via text (can't really do too much talking on the phone) and the next day I'm talking to uncle Stan and he says to me, "you might know already, Ya boy Randall; Slim died yesterday" I was "ahh man" "was it natural causes or was he killed?" "Covid got him" I said, "Wow, I was just thinking about him yesterday, that's crazy how I hadn't heard from him!" Slim was an old school playa from back in the days. Real cool cat had a lot of information he could bless you with because he has been around a lot and done a lot traveled everywhere and loved cars. I had this Rolls Royce Arnage he wanted to buy, "I'm waiting for y'all to bring the price down then I'm gon' come that car" he always said to me. "You sold the last one on me." We had another one he wanted to buy. He procrastinated and lost it. Good genuine dude, I'm going to miss Slim. We don't know when our time is up, we do know that we need to decide, and we know that we can't be in the guessing game when it comes to where our souls will end up.

One thing for certain, two things for sho' as Money would say; we are all going to die, and our souls are going to end up somewhere. Just sayin. I use a lot of words that might not be in the English dictionary and that's fine if you are not the judging type and even if you are.... thanks for purchasing and reading my book. I appreciate all that reading it! So many that are on their death bed with Covid, and their last words were, "I should've got the vaccine." I don't know how to take that. To me, that would be lack of faith or no faith at all and that's just my opinion and just like "booty holes' ' we all have those opinions that is, and I'm entitled to have mine just like you are entitled to yours. As I sit here writing I'm reminded that this was supposed to be complete the day I got released from the hospital. It did not work out that way, obviously I had more information to give Y'all and I'm ok with it. I always say, "I just want to be a blessing, then everything I need will be taken care of. "Facts! I hope you are enjoying it so far; I really do because it is just flowing out as I write. I mean just like a conversation with a million people or more. I know, sounds like wishful thinking, right? Well, it is more like speaking it into existence, being optimistic, knowing that it is predestined and in the cards if you will.

If I speak it, it will happen the same with negative. If you speak of negativity that's all you will attract is negative energy, people, and circumstances then you'll find yourself wondering why? That is not a good place to be, trust me I've been there where I would just complain about damn near everything daily from finances to not having enough clothes to a whole bunch of other dumb shit that really did not matter because guess what..I was still alive and healthy, so I could change all that as soon as I quit walking in circles and looked up and realized that I was walking in a freakin circle! See people can give you all the advice in the world if you don't use it to help yourself it is just a waste of their breath and time and that's unfair to them if you think about it, they don't think so though because they are genuinely trying to help you overcome this funk, you are in.

Truth be told there are not a lot of those people left since their children have now grown up and they don't have the same regard for life or others like we did back in our day, sad but so true. We're going to get it together though you guy's and it is going to get better in this world of ours .... Watch and witness we can't just keep going like this and letting the evildoers get away with all that they are forcing on us! We are much stronger, we serve a better God, we have no fear, we are smarter and "much" wiser. See we operate from wisdom, love, and know how, they operate from fear, hate and revenge. Who is going to expend the most energy based on the synopsis I just gave you? Well, think about it, if it takes so much energy to just wear a frown and you are not only wearing a frown you are also holding a grudge, fueling anger, plotting, and supplying anger with what it needs to feed your body so that it can respond to your feelings then the answer should be simple.... The evildoer! Years ago, I prayed for the spirit of discernment received it that night and it has been working for me ever since. "Thank you, Jesus!" There is this other thing that I acquired from my walk and relationship with the most-high. Whenever I feel the presents of the enemy or his minions, I say this aloud, "Satan I rebuke you with the blood of Jesus" and he must flee and leave me alone now, he can come back if he does with that spirit of discernment, I see him coming and I rebuke him with the blood of Jesus repeatedly however many times it takes eventually he gets tired and leaves me be. You have to say it aloud though, or it doesn't work. See, he doesn't have anything to do with your eternal soul. He can hear everything you say aloud. So, that's why you must say it "out loud."

I know people trip off some of the things I say and do like bending all the way down to the ground and picking an awkward box or object while keeping my head straight up so not to bend my back, or like when I was in the hospital screaming Hallelujah aloud because of the progress I was making, and I wanted to shout the highest praise to show my appreciation. I don't care what people think really, I'm going to do what I am supposed to do to fulfill my journey regardless of how I look or come across. That's your hang-up not mine so why should I concern myself with what you are choosing to allow you a set-back.

That would be stupid on my part. I can't control you or your feelings, behavior nor would I want to honestly. If I can't control it than it is not my fight just like when I was being impatient in the hospital wanting to get out there not now, but right now it was not my fight God had me, he told me so, I had to chill, relax, and let myself get better however long it took. Look at me now!

Wake up beautiful people! It's another day and if you are still reading my book then that means you are alive too! Congratulations, we both made it! I did not get a lot of sleep last night because I was binge watching this series called, "Safe" on Netflix. It was very intriguing and it kept my attention all night long. I will not tell you what it is about, I will tell you the executive producer is, Michael C Hall (Dexter) and he has a British accent in the series. You should check it out sometime. I think you'll enjoy it.

Woke up this morning feeling good, breathing was cool, coughing was minimal, so I decided to attempt five push-ups. One exhale, two exhale, three exhale, four exhale, 5 exhale, then I just kept on going to ten! That felt good to my chest muscles! I'm so thankful and blessed you guys I really am. Have you ever just felt so good about your surroundings, your health, your relationship, your life, your future, your endeavors? I mean just everything? I don't think I've ever felt this way before in my life up until now. If you have never experienced this feeling, I pray that you have it at least one time in your life because it is incredible, and you will wish it on everyone just like me! I've always believed that life is what you make it, you don't live how you got to, you live how you want to. If you want a wealthy life, then live like a wealthy person would, not like a "want-to-be" wealthy person would. Get to know some wealthy people. They are regular people just like us who decided to step out on faith, take a leap and landed on their success.

If you want a good life, well, I don't really have to say anything here that is self-explanatory about what needs to be done to accomplish that task. So, don't just sit and bitch about the things you wish you had or what someone else has, get off your ass and make something happen or you'll just be where you are. There are so many people afraid of being successful. Why is that? Dude! I just stretched and yawned at the same time, it has been so long since I've done that! I love appreciating the little things life has to offer. I am detail oriented like a mo'fo right now…. Lol!

Watched the Seahawks game yesterday afternoon. How disappointing, I think if we don't put some protection around Russell Wilson, we are going to lose him it is ridiculous how much he gets sacked right now! Why can't we ever have a good "O" line? It is what it is and I'm no fair-weather fan so, I reserve the right to get pissed at them if I want! Anyway, off that. Two thousand eighteen Q, me and D went down and watched the Hawks beat the forty niners for Monday Night Football, that was a blast! So many tailgate parties, it was bananas. The people were cordial. I mean you had some die-hard fans that got a little mouthy. We were just there to enjoy ourselves, they did not bother us at all, we had an agenda to get the "W" and get back home! Well, they are going again this year and obviously I can't go and that's sucks! It's cool though get stronger, and better than I was and maybe, I'll go to the Super Bowl or something if the Hawks make it. Don't ever count us out, Russell Wilson is our quarterback and Tyler Lockett and DK Metcalf are two of the best receivers in the NFL.... Just sayin. Great news! Maybe not to you, I'm going to tell you anyway since I do have your undivided attention.

My weight is coming back, and my stomach is still flat, well not flat, flat it is not pushing my shirt out at the bottom. I think I'll attempt another ten push-ups today to see how that goes plus there are some twenty-pound weights I can start on to do some curls. I'm set! What better way to recover than to work on my muscle mass at the same time?

I told you guys I'm coming back smarter too! This is no time for wasting time. This is high time for "plan your work and working your plan" – Gordon Montgomery (and old boss of mine) the first time he said it in a conversation we were having, I thought it was so profound, it stuck in my head because it made so much sense and it was simple words with a HUGE and thought-provoking meaning. I've put in song's and been quoting it ever since he said it to me in nineteen ninety-seven.

When I hear things that make me think about them while I'm listening to them, they get backed up in a mental data file that I used when I deem it necessary. I think that's where my wisdom is achieved, learning from someone else's mistakes and their experiences and applying it to my walk in and my journey.

This is so sad, this past weekend there were innocent bystander's lives lost because cowards just know how to pull the trigger instead settling their differences like "real men" do; with a conversation or if it comes to it, "fisticuffs" you live though no one must plan a funeral, moms don't have to be sad and distraught, your family don't have to seek revenge, there is no freakin war going on in the streets, children don't have to grow-up without a dad.

I mean a whole lot of positives on the opposite side of your decision to "take a life" FUCK!!!!!! The cops stop killing us because we are not having it anymore now, our own kids, our youth that we raised (not good and obviously not with God in the forefront) our killing each other and anybody else in the line of fire! I know of three dead and six wounded and get this, the two that I had the confrontation with..., they left the scene in separate vehicles and they both shot into the crowd in the parking lot and that's how they killed and wounded those people.

I knew the three that got killed, I knew the mom and the brother of the other two.

It hurt me inside my soul when I say that I mean my soul was sad and hurt and disappointed in us as a people and I just kept saying WHY, WHY?

I don't get it, I want to help, I want to do something

I don't want to be the "why" guy! I want to get on the front lines and help figure this thing out!

I know it is a spiritual warfare, I know and that's why God took the time to get me rested for the battle!!!

I have a song that I'm going to release called: "Try Some Black Love"

Here are the lyrics to the song:

We are strong people

We are smart people

We are tough people

And

We are not to be underestimated

We are congratulated

But y'all

We are becoming extinct

Cause

We're killing our own kind

And

That don't make no damn sense to me

We're not being rational at all

We are hunted, trapped and killed

We are running out of time

We are blowing our chances to be

Relevant up in here

We are dying at the hands of

Racist and

The police

We are black and brown

And

Many colors

So

Instead of killing each other

Why don't we just

LOVE US Yeah

Why don't we spread some

BlackLove

It's spiritual

It's powerful

It's from the heavens above

Why don't we just

LOVE US Yeah

Why don't we spread some

BlackLove

It's spiritual It's powerful

It's from the heavens above

BlackLovE

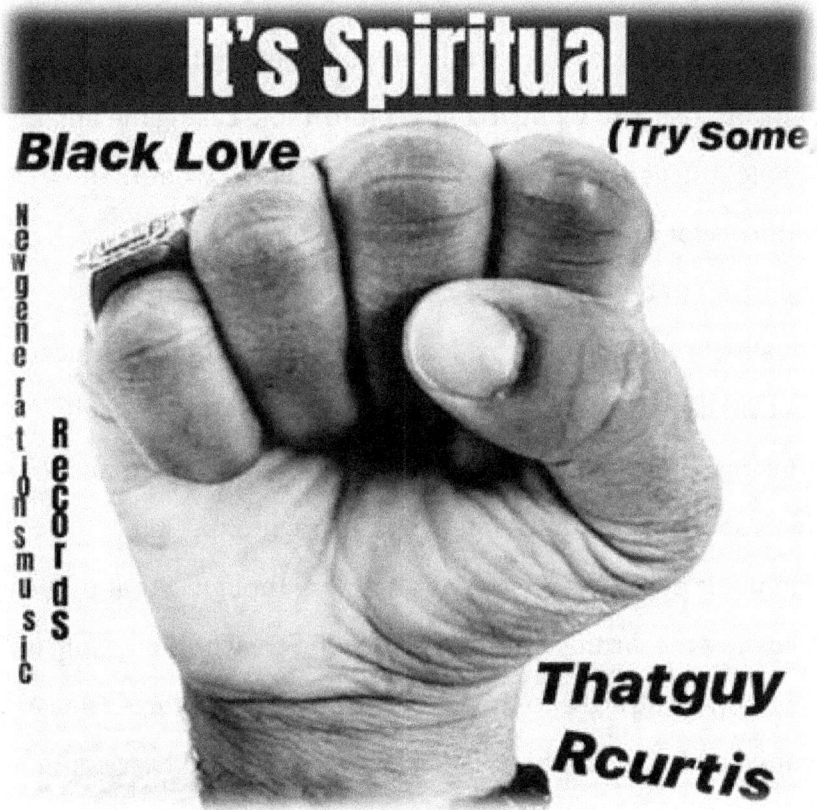

I'm listening to "BlackLove" as I am writing and feeling it all through my spirit and my soul, I just want to shout from the highest building with the loudest megaphone, "STOP THE NONSENSE DON'T YOU KNOW WHO YOU BELONG TO, DON'T YOU KNOW YOU ARE ROYALTY, DON'T YOU KNOW YOU ARE SEALING YOUR FATE???!!!" Black people or African Americans the chosen term for us this decade…. Lol. I laugh because who gives whoever the right to just change any race to any name they want?

I'm black bottom line! You don't get to change the name of my ethnicity to what you are comfortable calling me and my people, the gall, and the arrogance! You know what that confirms for me is this is not where me and people are supposed to be, you should not have to fight so hard for equality in your own home, it should be a given until you lose your privileges, there never should have been a white only drinking water fountain or a white only establishment and there should never have been white hate groups; KKK, skinheads etc.…. What they don't realize though is that they are following the wrong leader because who they are following is taking them straight to the lake of brimstone and fire! They are being bamboozled into thinking they got it made, how could you think as a human being that there are other human beings that don't belong here and that you and your kind are the only ones that are supposed to be on American soil, how do you sleep at night pleasantly wake in the morning with that same attitude and behavior??? I don't get it, nor do I want to. If we are being honest, I mean go back into the real history honest us colored folk built this land for you weirdos true you dictated and took all the credit because at that time we were your slaves and considered your property so, I guess by your laws and man-made up rules you had every right to do that. Now your plan is to try to eliminate us and poison us and mate our people with yours so that our black blood will become weakened and eventually obsolete (this is done by the power of suggestion tv, advertisements, social media) now I'm not angry or anything like that you do recall me saying if we are going to be honest well, that's what I'm doing.

So, like I said I'm not angry, how would that help the situation? It would not. I would just be another angry black person going through blaming instead of doing, another statistic instead of an activist and being an activist is just that, acting instead of talking, making moves instead of sitting still and doing nothing, having faith, and doing the work. I am fed up though, I am sick and tired of being sick and tired! I do have plans to make a difference, I will be heard and there will be change, souls will be saved, and those souls will save even more souls. Evil will not prevail, and HATE is I think the evilest you can be. Let's do it together regardless of your color, race, creed or even religion (which also is man-made) let's just "DO THE RIGHT THING!"

I used to look at demonstrations and see "White Americans' ' in them and I judged, I would say they are just there to be in something, they don't know the struggle, they are just collecting some bragging rights. At any given time, they can go right back to "White America'' and be forgiven and accepted back into their "white privileges! That was so wrong on several diverse levels. Who was I to make that assumption and more importantly, why was I making this my business, why did I overlook the problem and the reason for the demonstration and make that the new cause?

I tell you folks our brains our heads will have us in another dimension, space, and time if we are not careful. Needless to say, that doesn't happen anymore. I stick to the script if you will, especially now I have no time for negative energy and I know I have said it earlier in the book that lets you know how serious about this I am. We are on this subject, tough Huhn? This is where the spirit leads then we go with it.

My mother has had her home for forty plus years; paid for in the central district of Seattle Washington. How is that because "they" (we'll use that term because it's very fitting considering we don't know who the hell they are) decided "they" wanted the property that is now too expensive for the black people who have been there as long as my mom has. Now mind you the property is already paid for twice over. So, since "they" couldn't bully them out of their property "they" raise the property taxes so that these retired elderly black people on a fixed income can't afford to stay in the house they practically built. Gentrification, how come that's legal? Isn't that like a corporate hostile take-over, which is just bullying at the corporate level, and don't we teach our children bullying is wrong? You know "they" have a lot of hypocritical ways and "they" just get away with it. If "they" feel threatened "they" can shoot to kill you and it is justified, "they" can take your property if you don't pay the taxes that "they" make up, "they" can even put a lien on your property for a water bill! "They" are a powerful organization!

I wonder how come "they" don't do nothing for our homeless problems, I wonder if "they" family is safe? Hell, I wonder if one of "they" will read my book and get saved.... Lol! That sounds funny y'all know I don't put anything past God! We will find out after whomever "they" exploits "they "selves. This subject sucks! I should not even have to take up any of my precious time concerned about any of this. If this is truly "my home" I should feel safe and secure in "my home" country. I don't think so, it is filled with too much evil. So, I will do my part and when I'm finished, I know I have a home where I will be safe and secure and loved in Heaven.

I will not apologize for going on that tangent, it was called for. Someone is now enlightened and motivated and ready to get to work! I will say this, if you are planning on fighting for this or any other cause take your creator with you don't try to do it alone you need a higher power to protect your life you may get a few scrapes and bumps you'll still have your life though. If you have not heard or listened to anything else I've said in this book. PLEASE take that with you, store in a spot in your spirit that no one can touch "it will, save your life."

I got a treat yesterday; I was able to hug my grandbabies and my daughter for the first time in about a month and a half! It was great. I love them so much and anytime I can see them and spend some time with them is cherished! Having a relationship with my children and my grand babies means the world to me because it allows me to help with the raising of Nai Nai and Geno (my grand babies) and these day's that is so important with all these mis-guided kids on every drug that's available and the music being their new school sending the total wrong message, it takes a village like it always has the difference now is the village is living in fear of the children. Well, that needs to change! How do you live in fear of what you created? So, I am calling on, preachers, leaders, all races, creeds, color, gender, color, religion, politician, and anybody else that has any power to do something!

"Don't talk about it, be about it!" The only way there is change is when you make it. What are we waiting for?

Social media is making us more immune to the killings, like it's normal and we are going for it. I don't see too many people getting angry enough to say, "enough is enough" and that's what needs to happen!

WordStar, Facebook I don't know what other social media that's out there displaying grueling violence. I got sent something in my Facebook messenger somewhere in the middle east, a man being filet, alive, and then another where a man getting beheaded alive and aware! I mean that's not normal behavior, that's not something I nor you or anybody for that matter should be ingesting into our mental or more importantly our spiritual psyche. That's the world we live in, and right now it is seeming like it is by choice especially since there is no protest about it. The Devil is real y'all and recruiting on a daily maybe minute basis. That I don't know.

Answer this though, and put this in your mental Rolodex; if you knew you were going to a place that was going to be lonely, miserable, and so far under the earth that there is no telling what's down there (creature wise) would you want to go through that alone? If you are truthful and real about it, your answer will be "no" so there it is he is not wanting to go at this alone he is lying, promising, convincing and whatever he must do to get you to sell your soul to him and join him at the end of this whole thing in HELL! If you do not have a relationship with the most high you are in danger because you have no protection, you have no guidance, you have no savior.

The bumper sticker said, "If you're living life like there's no God, I hope you're right."

How profound is that? No judgment, lightweight rooting for you, even in that statement there is love being shown, no bashing, no negativity, just straight to the point and brief. Like I told you guys in the beginning of this book, you are going to hear a lot about God, Jesus, and the Holy Ghost. These are my beliefs, and I am not trying to force any of this on you, that's not godly if he gives us free-will who am I to take it away? I just am in love with the relationship that I have with him is all.

Thank you for not judging me.

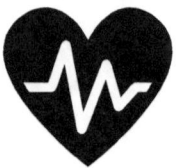

CHAPTER FOURTEEN

think I did too much yesterday, I got to try to take a little easier on myself with my current condition while recovering from Covid. This is no joke, this Covid needs to be respected. Anything that is created to kill you needs respect. It only has one mission so, it is focused and if you slip up; you are done, dead, passed away. I've seen too many dying from this evil disease and I could have been one too. I'm one of the chosen few, I've known that and felt some type of way my whole entire life, I just did not understand or know how to tap into it. Well at fifty-six years old I'm tapped! It doesn't matter my age, what matters is that I finally got it and now I can be used to complete my purpose in this life that I have been given a second chance to live.

There are two separate ways a person can respond to a life-threatening event that I had with Covid, one you can look it appreciate it and be thankful you are still alive or two, you can look at it as if you are invincible and you made through that no problem so, now you are just a bad man and can't nobody touch you! There are people out in our world that feel that way and carry themselves that way; Like fifty-cent – Curtis Jackson brags on being shot five times and living, the late Tupac Shakur bragged about being shot five times and living (RIH) and there is a few more that have bragged. Be thankful that you are still here and ask what it is you can do to show your gratitude. It might not be anything just let folk know I (God) brought you out the fire and made you better and for others it might be a little more involved it just depends on your calling and your original assignment. Mine is a little more involved and I'm ready for it!

There is so much talent in the graves because people did not utilize them while they were alive and because of that some people who are still alive were supposed to receive some information from those type people they missed out and did not get the information they needed to continue their journey the way it was planned out. I don't want to be one of those people, I want to leave empty, and all used up, I want to be so much of a blessing that the attitude I have carries over to my grand babies and their children and their children's children! I hope that it starts a movement so strong that everyone benefits from it and becomes a way of life!

See, "I had Covid And, it hurts"

Thank you for reading my book, I hope and pray that you got something out of it. This was a pleasure and I'm humbled and honored to be a vessel for your improvement.

God's blessings upon every one of you in Jesus' name. Amen!

Patience is indeed a virtue, and it sets apart the weak and the stronger. Patience can be tricky too, be careful if you are requesting it because it can last as long as you are alive and I don't think any of us want that it is usually just a certain situation or unfortunate circumstance that we need the patience for so, make sure you are clear when you are requesting patience.

Good morning it is about six forty-five in the morning, and I'm at it yet again. Today is ``Thatguy Rcurtis Show '' day and I have not been able to host it in over a month. My assistant is doing a superb job though in my absence. I'm very thankful to her! It takes a lot for someone to step-up at a moment's notice and pick-up where you left off. That's when you know, "this is what I'm supposed to be doing" this is in the plan.

Awesome!

Breakfast; turkey and egg croissant and tea... mmm, mmm delicious for my tummy Lol! Yes, I am taken care of on a daily basis; not bragging just testifying. Amen.

Today I gotta take it easy, I think I've been doing a little much physically. Yesterday was not a good health wise for me I got through nevertheless we made it through, and I got a surprisingly good comfortable night sleep. Yesterday though it was because I'm weaning off the steroids, I had a headache like I've never had before it was excruciating from my neck to my temples to my eyes. Natasha was like that's a migraine headache. Well, y'all know how I am. I'm not accepting that, so I said I don't get migraines and then I rebuke it with the blood of Jesus. I was not excepting that into my spirit! Got that right out of there…., pronto! I have never had a migraine in my life and I'm not about to start at fifty-six years of age.

I woke with no headache, clear nasal passage, and no coughing. So, yes, I will take it easy today.

Tomorrow is my first follow-up appointment sense I've been out the hospital; it is the soonest they could see me in, and it is cool because it gave me the opportunity to heal better and more expeditiously than normal so, now I can go in and they can see the progress and give me another month or two and release me back to the "hustle bustle" this life has to offer. I'm excited to get back in and go to work! Don't worry, I'll be calling on you guys for your support and you'll come because you'll see that these are not just words this is a manuscript a blueprint, if you will of a man who has had his life threatened by the evil disease Covid and survive to tell his story and dig in with his testimony. I never know what I will produce next because it comes through me for you so, I just wait get the info and off I go. I did with my promotions, the managing of bands, my "Domino for Breast Cancer" tournaments, now "Thatguy

Rcurtis Show" my talk show developed the day the mandate in Washington State hit, March 2020 and I've been rolling ever since. I need to produce a better time slot though because five o'clock pm pacific standard time is not a good "live show" time. I don't think it gives people a chance to wind down after work and prepare for the show. I'm still in thought about it. I'll know by January 2022 that you bet on!

Well, I've invited friends and family to meet my betrothed. They met her via phone while I was in the hospital; she was keeping them updated on my progress. I wanted to make sure they met the woman who sacrificed her life and health to take care of me and early in the relationship. Who does that? One who is hand-picked for you, that's who. Hand-picked, this is what was told to me while in prayer one day from that day I just ask for guidance on how to make sure I do my part in this thing: that's important to me. Not that I owe her for what she has done for me because truth be told, I would have done the same and she knows this. I just want to be all that I can for her from the beginning to the end and there is absolutely no way I can do that without his divine guidance. I'm not that savvy nor smart plus the woman species is extraordinarily complex and I'm not even interested in knowing how they operate or understanding them. Just want to know how to do my part and keep her smiling and wanting me.

I have now been out of the hospital as long as I was in on this Sunday, and I am so thankful!

I can remember being in that bed and barely being able to breath on my own. In fact I was on one hundred percent oxygen for the first week so, I was on life support. Then I remember them saying, "ok, we're going to move it down to eighty-five percent" I was thinking yes, I'll be going home soon. The next day one of the Doctors came in and said our goal is to get you down to four percent consistently then we can consider sending you home. I was just as cooperative as a military private, yessir ma'am or whatever. I just did not give anybody a tough time because I wanted out of there ASAP!

I was the best patient they had in a long time. A few of them were shocked when asked how their day was going, they did not even know how to respond and when I asked them if they heard me, they would say oh, were you talking to me? I'm not used to patient's asking me how I'm doing or being nice. Wow! How do you do that, how are you being a jerk on your possible "death bed?" "Well, get used to it when you come in here, because I appreciate everything you all are doing for me.

God bless and enjoy the rest of your day" is what I replied with. I made sure the atmosphere in my room was pleasant and peaceful regardless of a nurse with a nasty disposition; it did not matter; I was on a mission to get well and get out! "You get more flies with honey than you do shit" this is true if you don't believe me, do a little experiment of your own, record it and send to my email: aasdpublishing@gmail.com seriously, I'm curious to know who will take the challenge.

See, life doesn't have to be so serious all the time. We can make up our fun things to do and not focus on the "unwelcome news' ' and the turmoil, obvious issues and the craziness that is this life's state right now. So, breathe in your nose and out your mouth slowly five times, relax, thank your creator for another day, smile, encourage yourself with some positive affirmations, drink some water, and then get on with your day.

"Help me Holy Ghost!"

When I don't know my next move or how I'm going to make my next move this is what I say, and I was not sure what to write next in this book. There it is my secret, it is out now oh well, you needed to know... Lol! These little gems I'm blessing you guys with. I hope you use them because they are enormously powerful against all the adverse situations we must deal with on a daily basis.

SWITCH!

I have these two fingers that have been in sleep mode (numb) since I've been home. Well, now it's just the one. Man, it's really irritating to have a numb finger every day of the week. It feels weird. I tried banging it and stretching it. That's how I got the one finger to wake up this baby finger on my left hand though I am not having it. I do remember hearing folk talk about their leg or arm being numb all the time and I thought that would be a trip to deal with it, I was right it is a trip to deal with you gotta do what you gotta do. Can't let anything or anyone enable you from your duties or mission. NOT NEVA! That is what distinguishes a leader from a follower. Now, the best leader is a good follower; however, the difference is leaders follow successful leaders and followers just follow the crowd or whatever is in style. Us leaders have our own style. Which one are you?

This is my invitation to artist that wish to have their music played on: "Thatguy Rcurtis Show" (see the image at the last page of the book)

Ok, life, I'm back! Had to eat and take care of some administrative work, promoting and such. I look at my life and I feel blessed and highly favored because I have done quite a few things that I could be written off for and yet God still sees fit to carry me, protect me, cover me, give information I need to ward off demons, save me, wake me up for another day, give another three hundred sixty-five days to do it better and love on me. He gave me a singing voice, musical talent, the gift of writing, song's, poetry and now books. like "Lil Duvall" said, "I'm living my best life" and I ain't got time to waste on you neigh-sayers just watch my progression and stay mad. This is the time to do whatever it is that you have always wanted to do without any fear, go wherever it is you want to go without fear, say whatever it is you want to say without fear, help whomever you can without expecting anything in return.

The meek shall inherit the earth that's in the informative book, B-asic I-nstructions B-efore L-eaving E-arth. I'm sure it is the same in the other guides as well, just translated differently. We are at the end of these thoughts, of mine. I just want to take time to thank you all for reading my book and like I said I hope somebody gets something useful out of it. It was brought through me to you so, I did my part, and it feels tremendous!

Let's keep this going, let's help one another, make the best choice for our fellow human beings, let's refuse to hate, let's despise violence, let's build up our communities and let's always keep the creator first.

Let's build each other up, let's encourage each other on a daily basis, let's be cordial to each other on purpose and let's pray for one another. Let's not live-in fear, let's know that we are covered by the blood of the lamb and therefore the enemy does not have permission to kill us; he can mess with us all he wants though. Let's love and love and love some more on each other, let's speak whenever we walk past one another, let's figure out some way to avoid any kind of dictatorship and let's protect our children and grandchildren. Let's raise leaders and not followers, let's educate our children on morals, respect, loyalty, honor, dignity, and God's love. Let's go back to the village helping us raise our little ones as long as we do it through God our children will be safe. Let's go back to saying a prayer in the school's why not? That way we will have help fighting off the evil spirits and our children will not have to deal with so much and will enjoy life. What say you? "We have got to stand up for something or we'll fall for anything." Aren't you tired of children having to act like and be (light weight) treated like little grown-ups due to what they are having to deal with in this world that we let happen? I know I am and I'm not in the least bit interested in just letting it keep going. Getting angry is one thing, getting angry and following through is a completely different thing.

The children are the future and right now they are angry, confused, mental, hurt, scared, lost and that doesn't look like a good future representative to me. I wonder how many of us think about that. The future is going to be run by these children who have no regard for theirs or anybody else's life, they shoot first, they are on every drug known to man and they think that the way their living is the way they are supposed to be living. Wow, as I think as I write I'm like..., NO I have to do something, giving up on them is not the way! I feel like I should have titled this book, "What are we going to do about the children " because I'm really on the subject. It is very necessary, it is about time and don't play if you are about it then be about it if not, we would rather you not join. Your head must be right; your soul must be tight, and your spirit must be light there is no room for half-hearts you gotta be all the way SOLD OUT! This is serious business SO; WE HAVE TO BE SERIOUS ABOUT IT! Me having Covid and being in the hospital brought all this out. I would have never taken the time to even half-way think about any of this and that's a damn shame! I'm a little ashamed of making that statement and even more ashamed to know that it is true. See, that's where God comes in, he gives me rest, he is repairing me while we speak, and he is making sure that I'm stronger than I have ever been so that I can do the job he has for me to do.

Having Covid made me think long and hard on what my next three immediate moves would be as soon as I was able, book, music release and volunteer at the hospital for Covid patients.

Being in a position where your life is being threatened by a virus or trouble breathing is not a good feeling at all, you feel vulnerable and like I said before your head has you all over the place. I was one of the ones that made it through and I'm very thankful, there are a lot that I did not want to volunteer to see, perhaps if my spirit and experience can help create more success stories I will not know unless I try. None of God's people are supposed to die from this disease. I don't care what anybody says!

It can beat us down; it does not have permission to kill us!

Today's doctors' appointment went great although I was not under the impression that I still had the blood clot in my right calf. That's ok, I'm still alive and I'll be on blood thinners for at least six months. I will not be going back to work for about two more months and I'm good with that because I would rather go back closer to one hundred percent. This was my first meeting with this doctor. He was very thorough, and I like that he broke things down to me so I could understand what he was talking about, not a whole bunch of acronyms he used whole words! I think he will be my primary care physician since I don't have one, I seriously never got sick you guys, so I did not frequent the Doctors office.

My lungs are good, my heart is good, no wheezing in my breathing, my blood pressure and my temperature were great! So, overall, it was a successful visit plus I got to meet my new Doctor.

Today also was the day I gave my notice. I've gone to the platform that was hosting my show. As of October, six, twenty twenty-one (my mom's birthday) I will be independent, on my own, solo Dolo! Yes, watch me soar. My show is going to transform into something everyone is now talking about because of the content and the delivery as well as the entertainment!

"I aim to please and rarely miss!" That was the bumper sticker on my guy "Delaney's Capri" (RiH). That has stuck with me for over thirty-nine years, and it is a true statement as far as what I can guarantee about me. I don't know how to half-step, I only know how to give you what you want, entertain you how you like, and be the blessing that you need. So, trust me when I say to you, "Thatguy Rcurtis Show" you don't want to sleep on it. No exclamation points needed just a simple period to get the point across. Look you guys, if had not had to sit down with Covid I don't think I would be this motivated, spunky, focused, driven, ready to move forward on my journey I mean there are so many things to do that if I did not get this rest, I would not have the energy or the strength to do any of it. Case and point today in Tennessee at an elementary school a thirteen-year-old kid shot another kid and fled in a car he did later turn himself in. What reason did he have to attempt to kill another kid!?!? That's not it!

I HAVE GOT TO DO SOMETHING ABOUT THIS!!!!!!!!!!!!

AND I WILL!!!!!!!!!!!!!!!!!!!!!!!!!!!

CHAPTER FIFTEEN

I woke up this morning to "Killer Mike" who is a rapper and an activist and "Brother Louis Farrakhan" activist and profit. It was so powerful and uplifting and a confirmation for me as far as my mission for the extremely near future. These kids are killing kids and these rapper's advocate it with their lyrics and topics. It was amazing and strong; it was true, and no hold back. I loved it! All it did was motivate me even more to get to work! Here's the thing, ignorance is a bad and unhealthy behavior to have and display because this was my first time ever hearing Brother Farrakhan speak, I was listening to what other people had interpreted and just went with that. When I heard him speak this morning..., I was moved, and I appreciated his realness and his respect for God

Our world is not in a good place right now and if you think it is then you are in the twilight zone or outer limits because a world where the kids are getting rid of each other is bound to soon fade away into nothing. We are in a state that we must search high and low for some love, peace, and respect. It's not just readily available anymore. Folk rather be mean, standoffish, difficult, mad and distrusting that is many of our fellow human beings. How do you think we are going to last like that? We are not, the evil one will just take-over and reveal his face and all who have fallen for his tricks and promises will be carried off with him because he already bought your soul and there is no going back on this contract. So, man GET IT RIGHT now! It is up to you who you choose, since God is a just God, he will not force you to choose him he will, except you if you do though.

It's a challenge for me to breath without coughing to this day and I still see fit to say, "thank you Jesus and thank you father and hallelujah! You want to know why...? I'm ALIVE! So, if I have to work a little harder to breathe then guess what, I'll do the work, I'll fight that little fight because the battle has already been won!!! Most of you would be complaining you cannot breathe, tired of sitting home, really, I got a blood clot and whatever else you can find to whine about when you should be thankful for your life and a second chance. That's what I mean when I say, "take advantage not for granted" there is a significant difference between the two.

People, from here on out let's all be unique all of us who are reading this book let's be the unique crew. The crew that makes things happen, the crew that don't talk much, the crew that will beat you down with our intellect, the crew that is not scared of anything, the crew that spreads the truth, stands by it, and compromises it for no one or nothing. Let's do it! If you have made it this far, you are going to tell somebody about this enjoyable read. I'm writing it and reading at the same time, and I'm intrigued. We really don't know what we can accomplish until we can execute. Self-motivation is not an easy task; it comes with self-doubt, self-pity, self-absorption, selfishness, self-indulgence, self-recognition, and a few other adjectives that a lot will judge. Don't pay attention to them, they just wish they had the courage to do the same as you and stand up for what they believe in. Haters are people who don't even know who they are, so, since they don't understand how you could be so focused and driven all they can do is despise you, talk all kinds of negative things about you and just know you are doing something illegal, and you'll get caught soon enough. Whoever has that much energy and time to focus on what you are doing has plenty of time to soul search and get themselves together and do the same thing you are doing.

See, so they are not haters, they are simply confused kid adults with no role model…. Lol!

I just took a common complaint about a certain type of behavior of people and made it not so concerning then flipped it to a positive. It all depends what your priorities are, what you are focusing on and what is important and what is not so important. We can all do better in that respect.

For example, I tell my baby all the time, don't honk at people who cut you off or drive erratically because you never know what they're going through. Plus, it doesn't change anything but your mood for the day. Control it! Don't let it control you! The choice is yours. Make the right choice that is

going to benefit you, to hell with them and their attitude and
/or ignorance. You have things to do, plans that you have
made, and you plan to accomplish. So, tell me again what part
of your plans included that erratic driver? Exactly! We must
stay conscious of our every move, we must stay on our path
and walk around the boulders in the way, step over the big
rocks and kick the pebbles out the way then keep on moving.
We must control our feelings when we are on our mission
because the enemy is always going to toss in a diversion and his
little minions are going to try to trip us up along the way so,
stay prayed up, weaponed up, and uplifted! We have a
responsibility to be the ones to make the change happen by
whatever means necessary. Can't be no punk in this thing
better be all in or it will not work and any weak link in the chain
is going to render us all vulnerable.

Just think about all this because of my battle with Covid.

I was blind but now I see

Broken but now I'm repaired

Lost but now I'm found

Weak but now I'm stronger than I've ever been

"I Had Covid And, It Hurt's" to see what I've seen witness what I'm still witnessing and do absolutely nothing to help any of it and enjoy my life like it has nothing to do with me.

Something must give people

Cause…,

"This ain't livin" – Marvin Gaye

Here recently just a couple of days ago I was informed that a 77-year-old man took his own life. Now, what would possess you to do that? That goes to show us all "we never know what's going on with a person, just because it looks as though everything is alright. You would think that after many years of life a person would be thankful and feel blessed to have had the opportunity to be a blessing. You just don't know what is going through his or her mind at any given time. I was having dinner with some friends, and the question was asked if you give a person a chance or do you feel they must earn it?

I immediately said that I give everybody the chance to demote themselves; however, it comes with an "A" already. I used the analogy of the high school teacher's introduction: do the class work, test, homework, show up to class on time every day, you have an "A" whichever of these tasks you do not complete you will demote your grade. I think that's fair, so I adopted that concept in life and so far, it has been working.

My Nana (may she RIP), used to say, "respect is, do a dog" I never understood what she meant by that until much later in my life then when I got it, I applied it as well. If you are driving down a road and a dog hops out in front of your car, you are going to hit your brakes to avoid hitting the dog and you don't know this dog, you have never seen this dog before in your life; however, you would give him/her that respect. So, that being the case, why does your fellow human being have to earn your respect? To me, there is more energy wasted. Just let a person demote themselves; it doesn't even take long for them to do it.

Isn't it amazing the stuff you think about while you are sitting still and thinking about nothing? I mean it is like thoughts just find themselves in your brain and you begin to process them. Case and point; I had no intention on drafting a book, completing it, and getting it published. I was just planning to work on my music and "Thatguy Rcurtis Show" and that's it! Then along came a thought while me and silence were chillin' and here you have it a book. It is awesome though because I feel like I've been chosen to tell this story and tell it like no one else ever could! I accept the challenge and I thank you for the confidence.

Man, I wish I could play some "hoops" being on these blood thinners. I have to be careful because I'm vulnerable to bleeding out or even worse a head injury could cause me to hemorrhage. Oh, well at least I 'm alive. Oh, I just found out that while I was in the hospital my kidneys failed…, whoa! Never was none the wiser. It is best that I did not know in a way because I would have freaked out knowing that my kidneys failed. Like I said before, it is easy to get into your own head, it is better to reach into your soul and pull-out prayer. I knew I was going to be taken care of. I'm still human though. Most folks would have been sick and tired of being at home, not me. I'm enjoying the time with the family and getting things done that I should've done already. Music, my show and some other personal things. This is the time to take care of "me!" Not in a selfless manner in a manner that I can be the blessing that I pray to be on a daily basis.

So, we must take the time to achieve the goals we have for ourselves and whatever is in our spirit and has been in our spirit; neglected and put on the backburner because if we don't eventually, we will have some regret and I think that will create some type of anxiety. I'm not a doctor that makes perfect sense though. So, don't just be, be who you want to be and who you were born to be anybody can have a job with perfect attendance and a bunch of merits, it takes a special person to live their dreams and live well! I let's be honest, we all have dreams, not all of us work towards making them come true. The last thing I like to think about is if I did everything I was supposed to do within my life, if I said the right thing to whomever, if I taught someone what they needed to learn or if I testified to the folk I was supposed to testify to. My goal is to leave a legacy for people to learn from and grow from. I especially want to reach the children, the young people who are "out of control." . I know I cannot save all of them. Let's make a conscious effort to save some of them.

Money helps make the world go around and it helps with attempting to start a movement or create a cause. It is not easy to require when you are on that type of vibe though and it is cool…, whatever is meant to be will be no question. If you write a song and it is supposed to be heard by certain people or a particular person, it will be released and delivered, if you have a program or show that is teaching and supporting it will be successful, no doubt. So, be patient and wait your turn because it is coming sooner than you think, bet.

Every now and again I reflect on the fact that I was fighting for my life a little over a month ago with Covid and I trip a little bit because when I was in the hospital, I really did not think that way well, maybe..., a couple times, I was always saying, "it's not my fight, God got me" and I believed it wholeheartedly. You guy's if I would have given into my head for one moment it would have been curtains for me this Covid can do you in if you let it. No disrespect to any of your loved ones who passed away from this evil disease whatsoever, this is just my strong belief. To this day I still have issues with breathing, and I've been out of the hospital now for three weeks, I cannot walk too far, or I'll start coughing like crazy and I'll have to catch my breath. My strength is nowhere near a hundred percent. It is just, hurry up and wait. I was told that I have some type of long -term Covid not where I'm still contagious. I guess it means I will have some side-effects that will last for a little longer than normal you know me though; I'm not excepting that! I have way too much to do to be down for too long. By the end of this year, I'll be ready!

SWITCH!

Today is a quiet day for me. I don't want to say the wrong thing or come off arrogant or smart-assed. I just want to have a pleasant day. Yesterday I had a moment where I was told in my spirit to, "shut-up" and I did. It was a little weird. I still did it though because it was best. Sometimes we need to "shut-up" just because you have something to say doesn't mean it's the right place to say it. You could totally screw someone up that was not supposed to hear or absorb what you put in the atmosphere; we gotta be careful because everything is not for everybody. Once we get that down pat, we will have grown a little bit wiser.

I don't know if I said earlier or not, I put Thatguy Rcurtis Show on hold until January 2022 due to me recovering and not having to stress about the show, the guest, and mostly to not put so much pressure on my assistant. I figure I should have it all together by then and be able to operate more efficiently. You have got to make those executive decision and I feel good about it.

My music on the other hand I will continue to work, produce, release, and create while recovering because that is my solace. I have a few songs available now. I want to incorporate some other musicians with a couple of them to give them a little flair. I've never collaborated yet. I think it will be good if I can find someone willing. Most people don't look at me that way and that's cool because I met some different musicians around the globe that I can reach out to. One way or another I will get it done! Trust and believe that!

I'm gaining my weight back and my stomach is still basically flatter than it was, my butt is rounding, and my chest is forming. I just must get back to my push-ups when I can and sit-ups then I'll be good and stronger than I was. Dope!

I have a feeling that my singing is going to be better as well; cannot wait to see. I know my writing has evolved into something different. I'm excited about my future! I have a lot to share with you all and it is all good. If I told you I've learned quite a bit while recovering I wonder if you would believe me? It doesn't matter, I'm just sharing with you and eventually you will see what I'm saying to you in this book. You see, you cannot be spared a second chance and come back and be the same, act the same, live the same and praise the same. You must come back a changed person and "ready for that action boss" – Marshawn Lynch. I'm a giant, I'm getting my rest then I will have the strength needed to get to work. Not just selling cars; saving lives and souls. Amen. Got to go buy towels and linen now, I'll get back up with you guys later. Peace'

Man, yesterday I had a pain in my chest that disallowed me to move and barely breathe. I mean it was like the worst muscle spasm ever! I did some research because I wanted to make sure I was not having a heart attack and it turns out that me being on blood thinner medication saves me from having a heart attack; however, being that I'm recovering from covid, headaches, chest pains, coughs etc. Normal. Today, it is a little better, still tender and bothersome when I inhale. Wrapped it up with an ace bandage to try to take some of the pressure off and see if this will help some and it did, I'm not in the same pain as I was yesterday.

This is crazy and commendable at the same time. While we were out shopping for our linen and towels, I witnessed this white guy trying to steal a whole basket of merchandise from the store and there was this younger black man who stopped him from getting away with it. Now, while in the process of preventing the white man from stealing the merchandise the white man was trying to push this younger black man into striking him so he could have a lawsuit, what I was impressed about with this younger black man is he did not back down, and he did not let the white man take him out of his character and focus. The white was pushing him, and you know you are allowed to use the same force that another uses on you so, they got into a little shoving match and that was the extent of that. What I was impressed with is the fact that this younger black man did not knock this white man out for putting his hands on him, that showed a lot of restraint and discipline. Me, I don't think I would have had that same restraint, first you are all in the wrong and you got caught; take your losses and leave. Putting hands on me would have been open season on "knock out time". So, I'm immensely proud of that younger black man.

Here's the thing you guys, you can learn from any situation or any one person. I learned yesterday from that younger black man that you don't always have to" go ape" in a situation. Sometimes it is best to take the "high-road" in that case it worked out best for the younger black man because he did not jeopardize his job and saved himself from an assault. We got to be more conscientious of making sure we think before we react. Just saying.

You might be wondering why I keep specifying him as being a "younger black man" . It is because I want to stress to all my readers that our" younger black men" do know how to make the right decision to benefit themselves.

Today started out nice and once your morning starts off beautiful the rest of the day must follow. Great breakfast, incredible smiles invigorating conversation and it is just getting better as it progresses. Great football games today and I think I will be completed with, "I Had Covid And, It Hurt's" finally!

This has been a real treat and a challenge both to do (author this book) even though it is inspired by my father in heaven, I still must produce the things to say and the lay out and things like that. It has been fun too!

I'm very thankful to all of you for reading my book and like I said before I hope y'all get something out of it. Here is something that you don't think about everyday…, "sometimes love ain't enough" explain this Rcurtis.

MESSAGE!!!!

Ok, I will. I find that most people in relationships stay in them because there has been so much time involved or there's kids involved, or they feel like it might get better when they should just get out while they still have their sanity. Here is this problem. Say you have been in a relationship for five or more years it is easy to get stuck in a rut due to the years together; however, what about thinking more about you and your feelings and opportunities? Now I'm not suggesting that you just not give it your all or even try a counselor and I'm talking about when you have exhausted all the programs and chances and now you must love you more than you love this relationship.

There comes a time when you have to say, "enough is enough" and you have to get "sick and tired of being sick and tired" and move on. Now don't get me wrong I have a little bit of separation anxiety. I had to realize eventually it was time to take care of me and my emotions and feelings and allow myself the opportunity to get my happiness enhanced. So, that's what I mean by, "sometimes love ain't enough"

I forget who the preacher was that said this, "you can love from afar." After you make that decision and make that move forward you find that the love you had is just that, the love you had. You move on with a smile on your face and feeling a lot better about every day you wake up in the morning because there is no more arguing for no reason, fighting, waiting for some sort of compassion, passion or just some freakin companionship type conversation. Can you tell I've been through it… lol? I am no longer in that type of relationship because I finally decided to look out for myself and more importantly, wait on God to fill in the blank and the feeling is so awesome!

You know what? This is going to sound a little weird and some of y'all might even think there is something wrong with me. If it was not for me going through covid I might have lost this opportunity of this incredible relationship I'm in right now. I think you should always find a positive in everything you go through, be that it is good /or bad; the glass is always half full and never empty as long as you have something to fill it back up with. Life is easy you guys; we make it difficult by trying to go it alone.

God gave us this world to live in. If we ask him how we are supposed to live and what we are supposed to be doing while we are here, he will let you know individually.

I'm telling you what I know, not what I've heard.

We

Are

Here

To

Help each other

So, let's do it! We are all we got!!!

There is no limit to what we can accomplish if we try and plan for it. Most times we are our own worst enemy and we hold ourselves back from being successful. We are all designed to be happy, fulfilled, needless and satisfied. Those who understand that, get it, and go on to be whatever they want and do whatever they want to do. It is not easy to do; however, it is a lot easier than difficult.

I think encouraging our children and grandchildren to work for someone else's company is doing them a dis-service. Encouraging them to be entrepreneurs is the best thing we can do. Why teach them to be workers when we can teach them to be bosses and leaders and run their own company? Slavery was abolished centuries ago and we are still trying to keep it going with our teachings. Our future is not looking so good with the children we are witnessing today. A lot of them are murderers and drug addicts and mean confused scared human beings so that's what we must look forward to in our near future.

Not something to be excited about, right? Well, if that is the case, and that's the way you truly feel, then we need to do something NOW!

If we all do our individual part, we will be able to help our situation before it is too late.

Every day I wake up and I send my children and my grandchildren a positive and edifying message that they can take with them and utilize throughout their entire day. I do it on purpose so that they know they are leaders and not followers. Even as an adult's we sometimes need some type of encouragement to move forward and have the confidence needed to accomplish our goals.

Random acts of kindness. How often do you practice this wonderful gesture?

Don't worry, I cannot count either. I did reap the benefits here lately at a restaurant. The host asked if we were celebrating anything special and I blurted out "yes, we just got engaged" she said the customary congratulations and proceeds takes our drink order. When the drinks came, she said," these drinks are from the table next to you" I was shocked, didn't know "random acts of kindness" still existed in our world today.

So, we toasted, and we thanked the couple (married 30 years) chatted a little and of course I bought them a round we even exchanged information. Cool people. I know it was just drinks. It was still a nice gesture, thoughtful and genuine. That seems to be rare anymore in our society and that's sad. Imagine if that type of thing happened to us every day what kind of attitudes we would have throughout the week. Pretty positive and in a great mood, I think.

The reality is, we are not there yet due to so many other issues that are roaming around in our mist and in the wind. There again, it is up to us as individuals to make a difference. Is it strange to you how the common denominator to all our worldly problems is "us" as individuals? Well, it is, and it does make sense because we all have our own individual thoughts, way of doing things, process and timing therefore making it almost impossible for us to do it together. We would have to first get it down in our own heads and spirits then we could formulate a plan together at that time. Everything has a process and if it doesn't then there will be serious issues and it will not prosper. Let us use pro sports for example. Do you think if Pete Carrol did not have a plan and his staff did not follow his process the SeaHawks would win any games? Absolutely not! That sums it up, yes? Good!

My chest pain is subsiding and now I have another version of coughs! Man! It is a random cough, a little flem, no congestion, just a cough when it comes it continues for a little bit then it stops and makes me have to blow my nose. This sucks I mean really sucks! There are people who are sick all the time, in the doctor's office all the time, dealing with some sort of pain all the time and they just deal with it. I am dealing with it the best I can. The difficult part of it is being unable to move like I would normally move. How does a hypochondriac do it? I am not a fan of hospital's or just being out of commission. I must be active and productive. I don't know how to sit still and be a "bump on a log" so to speak. The crazy thing is, there are people like that, they are ok with doing nothing and sleeping from couch to couch, bumming, not having anything, not even able to afford their own habit, cigarettes, and such. Then when you try to help them, they just take you for granted. Who does that, how can you be ok with yourself with this behavior? Anyway, it is what it is I guess, and it is not for me to understand, nor do I want to. I just want to do what is meant for me to do and help who I am supposed to help, walk in my blessings and at the end get my reward of eternal life.

I am in my head right now as I write trying to figure out where to start writing and what to write about. That's funny because as I am writing…. Lol. We are some hilarious creatures!

My blood clot is still in effect, the doctor said it will be a while before my body dissolves it completely so, I am still on blood thinner medication. Got to be careful on those pills, anything can cause an unpleasant situation. I am ok with that. Taking it easy seems to be my new way of life these days. Just got a call from physical therapy. My doctor thinks I need to work on my motor skills, and I am just going with the flow and not being resistant at all for obvious reasons. So, I have an appointment tomorrow at ten forty am, gotta be there twenty minutes early for paperwork though.

Now it begins, the work involved to speedy recovery, the physical part I have been on the mental and the spiritual since I have been with and now recovering from this evil disease, Covid. You know what movie I watched the other day, and it reflected this pandemic to me. Just a little, "Outbreak." They developed a disease for chemical warfare, and it got compromised by a "jackass" and became a worldwide epidemic. Now, I'm not suggesting that this is the way that the Corona virus came about; however, I have always thought that certain movies depicted the way things will be in this world eventually, like look at "Back to the future" and "hoverboards" or futuristic movies and electric cars, phones that you can see and talk to people on, virtual reality coming to life now just to name a few. It is not too far fetched if you really think about it which we are far too busy to do; stop and think. Wow! Kinda deep, huh? I know, it is necessary.

Speaking of the future, why has customer service and caring for the client gone to complete "shit?!?!" I mean from the cell phone service at the grocery stores. Doesn't anybody train their employees anymore, conduct a class on good customer service? It is ridiculous! It has gone from, "may I help you sir or ma'am" to a head nod and a "what's up". Really? These are our children and grandchildren that are practicing these insanely horrible customer service antics! People, our world is going to perish, and it is on us, we are just tolerating all this crap and moving on like there is nothing to see or do here! Are you really ok with all of this?

Well, I am not! Not even a little bit! In fact, I am totally pissed about all of it! Watch, you'll see how pissed I am, and you will either join or remain a "Walking Zombie!"

Just existing until your decapitated, incapacitated and finally destroyed. If you are ok with that, I am not ok with you.

Stand UP for Something or Fall for Anything!

We need soldiers willing to fight for "us" and our future...........................

The KIDS!!!!!!!!!

The problem is we failed the system, we did not plan the work properly and we did not have the best process in place. We gave them too much power and they did not even know what they had. They took advantage of it though I think to this day kids are calling the police on their parent's. That is ridiculous that they have that kind of power but, that's what was wanted and here we are. How does it feel to now be afraid of the children that you bore into this world? I say you purposely because I'll be damned if I fear my seed! They are my responsibility, and I will not let them down! Fortunately, mine are now adults with their careers and their goals and they are doing well for themselves. My grandbabies are the reason I do what I do now and practice what I preach so they always have a leader they can depend on.

There are still strays out there with nowhere to turn, because how are you going to have respect for someone who fears you especially if it is your parents? As long as there is breath in our lungs, it is never too late! So, let's shut up together and figure it out before it gets out of hand and we must revise another plan, and another, until we decide to move forward with "the plan" FEAR doesn't exist, it is something we conjure up to make excuses to not have to do the work before us. We are Gods' children, therefore we don't have that spirit of fear in our beings, unless of course we invite it in.

We are powerful people when we think and then respond, we pray and then wait, we fight then conquer. We don't have to announce we are on route, we just show up ready. The only time the right hand knows what the left is doing is if the brain makes the right aware otherwise, it is none the wiser. Got it? Good! We possess a lot of power as I mentioned before, we just must tap into our "common Sense" and there it is. If you see a doorknob, don't try to break it down and figure out why it turns, just turn it, and walk in or out the door, common sense. So simple, so plain and powerful! We all have this power because we all have common sense; we all do not utilize it though and therefore some of y'all seem to fall short of your blessings.

Blessings are important in our lives because it's God's favor for us. So, if we don't acknowledge them as that, then we are merely existing and stumbling daily. Who wants to stumble at all? Certainly not I and I'm sure you do wish to stumble either, yet and still there are a lot of our fellow human beings who refuse to release their own judgment and self-accomplishments and place the credit where it belongs, to the one who gives us life and grants us grace and mercy. So, for that reason they continue to stumble and eventually fall short of their blessings.

Don't you think it is better to live a more peaceful and confident life?

I don't know about you, I for one am glad to have the relationship I have with my heavenly father, if it wasn't for him, I would have been lost in the jungle of self-pity, self-doubt, self-destruction and self-caused suicide. Being in your head all the time will cause an abundance of stress and pain which will lead to anger and hate which I'm sure you can agree is not good for the mental capacity of your brain. Mental health is real, and no one understands it better than a person who has gone through it and survived. I bet you if you asked a person who has survived a mental health crisis who they must thank for their survival they will undoubtedly say, "God."

I am who I am and all I know how to be is me. If you are not cool with that I understand and respect it. The problem with most people is they try to be something they are not to impress someone or some one's who are not even worth it. That is too much energy wasted on nothing. So, don't do that! Just be you and be satisfied.

Another thing, women stop with the thirsty photos on social media all you are going to get is a man or (these days) a woman who is going to quench your thirst then leave you dehydrated, and you will be right back where you began because that's what you advertised; give me something to drink and you are in to win it! Unless of course that's what you want.

Men, y'all need to start showing these ladies respect so that they can start respecting themselves. If y'all let them know that the way they are presenting themselves is not acceptable then the lot of them will change. Some of them want a good man, they just do not know how to wait for one and they have the wrong concept on how to attract a good man. Y'all portray women as sex objects beneath you and that's not why God created her. He created "Eve" to be our "help-meet" not our sex slave or any other derogatory title or adjective we can think of. Can't make a "hoe" a housewife and why would you want to? Now, here is the thing at the same time..., that housewife can be neglected, disrespected, abused, and lose herself in a state of confusion and try "hoe" on for a stint. Our women are delicate creatures, and we must treat them as such.

Anymore there are no boundaries, and anything goes; however, we must protect our women and let them know we love and appreciate them. Now, I am going to say something, and it is not to offend. I really think that some of our women, especially our black queens, turn to each other for love because good black men are rare anymore and some of them are on the downlow. Society could be blamed but, at some point in time we must take responsibility and change the trajectory ourselves. See, although it is not a fair playing field, we as black people must figure out how to work together and make sure our children and grandchildren are not in the same vein as it is these days. They deserve a chance to make their own decision and choose their own path.

Confession time.

I have two children, and both have decided to be with the same sex; daughter with a woman and my son prefers men. So, you see I cannot be prejudiced or anything of that nature. I genuinely am a little curious though as to why.... and not just my children but in general? I will never get that answered and to be honest it is not that important it is just a query of mine. I love my children first, whatever lifestyle they choose is their decision and I respect it. My daughter always says,

"Love is love."

I really do not know where this page of the book came from or why all I do know is everything is for a reason and sometimes we do not find out why until it is time to find out why, other times we might not ever find out why due to the fact of it not being for us at all; we are just being used to pass along the information.

You know how when you were taking the SATs in school and the teacher would always say go with your first answer and don't second guess yourself? I normally would go back through the page and re-read and correct any thing I thought did not sound right or look right on this page, and for some reason I am not going to do that, or should I say these pages because now it has migrated into two pages. My son gets mad at me when I say that it is a choice he made. He believes he was born this way and who am I to argue so, I do not because it is insignificant to me my thing is to respect and love my son. This life is too short for that to be a hang-up on either one of our parts, in my humble opinion.

Life is too short to have any hang-ups honestly. Someone you do not like for whatever reason, should be forgiven or totally left alone. A relative you are beefing with should be forgiven and the issue forgotten and then move on. If you have a parent and for some reason you have not talked to them in years or days because of a misunderstanding or an argument you had; apologize and move on, unless it was life-threatening it is not worth it; there will be a void in your life, your head, and your soul. Think about it, and then fix it.

I had Covid And It Hurt because it made me reflect and contemplate. I must be with myself and make some serious life changing decisions. Having Covid made me look in the mirror and forgive myself and deal with the fact, I could have been one of the ones that did not make it out of the hospital alive.

Having Covid has brought this book to life for a reason and only the ones that this book is for will know the reason.

I believe this is going to be another way to be that blessing that I consistently request to be. I'm enjoying writing this book and the fact that I already know what the next book is going to be about is half the battle.

Woke up this morning to a new day and I thank God immediately because I'm happy to be alive and getting healthier by the day. My lungs are not as strong as they should be, and my strength is not a hundred percent either. I'm taking it slow though.

It's important to take it slow because it is possible to relapse, and I do not want to be back in the hospital any time soon. Don't get me wrong I'm grateful for all that they did within their power to help along in the process. I'm just not a hospital type guy. I never have been so, I'm nowhere near interested in being a patient any time soon.

Having this evil disease had opened my eyes up to a lot of essentials like, brushing my teeth on my own, waking up and walking down stairs, cleaning my room, washing my own clothes, cooking a meal, taking out the garbage, vacuuming my rug I mean simple things that we typically take for granted, I can't mow the lawn yet and that's a drag I will be able to soon enough though. I want to hoop so bad!

I think I may have referenced that earlier in the book that's how bad I want to. I miss the stage too! Singing with the band, controlling the crowd, having a blast! Well, I must come to grips with the fact that this is my next chapter of my life like it or lump it. Everything that takes place in my life now must be a benefit and forward progress or I can't fool with it. No time for wasting just positive energy and profitable moves.

When I say profitable, I mean, physical, financial, spiritual. It's not all about the money for me, I get excited when someone else wins because of my energy and or words of wisdom. Remember, I just want to be a blessing? So, if you meet me or know me then you know what to expect of me because when I say that and especially when I pray for it best believe I mean it with all my being! You know what though you guys, it is not the easiest thing to do because people are typically not cool, they're jerks, mean, evil, selfish, nosey, and filled with drama.

In my travels and I find I really must rely on the weapon God provided me with which are these words: "Satan I rebuke with the blood of Jesus" I'm telling you if you believe it works, it doesn't make you invincible it will be a temporary fix. We are not ever going to be perfect, only God is. We will go through somethings, and we will get angry and slip up because we are only human..., don't take that for granted though or that will make you weird as the rest of the people. Every one of us has a purpose in this life and it's up to us as individuals to tap into what it is and start working towards it. The thing is, you don't have to if you don't want to; "free will" , who else's God says that? You don't have to serve him if you don't want to; I'm always here though.

That was rhetorical.

I believe you get my drift.

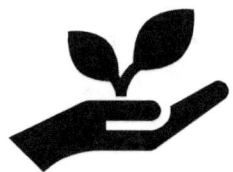

CHAPTER SIXTEEN

This is something that I have always wanted to do, and it took much needed rest for me to pursue and get it done.

I am glad that I finally decided to author the book because while writing I was able to dig a little deeper into myself and appreciate the silence because it allowed me to grow in mind and spirit.

I hope you were able to get something out of anything I said in this book.

My goal is to be that blessing that I pray to be daily.

This is not a selfish attempt to get any selfless gratification, this is an attempt to start my mission to help others become and do what they wanted to always do and never took advantage of the opportunity.

Only you can get yourself over that hump and DON'T BE AFRAID OF SUCCESS!

There are many reasons to want change and there are even more reasons to want to change. If we investigate our own selves, we will be able to find what it is that we need to change. Blaming others or judging other's is not the answer because when you point one finger the other four are pointing at you.

Our world is in desperate need of a make-over, we are not acting civilized, we are hating more than loving, fighting more than loving, killing more than loving. I know that is not what is expected of us.

This man-made emotion called "pride" has taken over our complete passion and compassion for one another and made us think that the way we are is ok. Well, it's not and it's also teaching our children both young and old to do the same. We must STOP IT now! Look at the future potential.... bleak and very violent!

I for one refuse to just sit back and let it happen, I will get my hands dirty, if need be, just so that my grandbabies and their grandbabies can have a chance at a better way of life.

This book is only one of my works and ways to make as many people as possible aware of the detrimental effects of not trying to adjust to the majority of all the chaos and dilemmas we're suffering from right now.

If we decide to just sit idle and do nothing that is exactly what our future will be and amount to; nothing.

So, what say you, are you willing to just do nothing or are you ready to start the work needed to make a better place for all of us?

This is not an overnight answer nor is it an overnight success. This will take as long as it takes, so you will have to be a soldier willing to fight until the battle is won!

Nothing beats a failure, but a try – Granny GG

If it wasn't for my faith in God and my relationship with him, I never would have made it out of the Covid jungle.

With the mental complexity of trying to stay, there (in reality) there is no chance of making it without a higher power.

This might seem repetitious. That's fine obviously. It needed to be repeated for someone. I have no problems reiterating when necessary.

Right now, you are probably saying to yourself or even out loud, I thought the book was done already. And it is, just consider the after effects, the last part, the remanence of a good word or words, the rest of the end. I don't know, call it whatever you want or just accept it for what it is. Yesterday is a memory, tomorrow not promised today is an opportunity to get it right and on a daily basis that is the plan.

I know why I survived Covid. I'm one of the chosen few. I'm supposed to get a lot done while I'm here. I know that might sound strange to you and it's supposed to unless you are one of the chosen few as well.

Before Covid I didn't make time for myself to bring the gifts out of me that were and still are in me so, it was time to either start or die. I know that sounds harsh and to say it I was a little hesitant. I have plenty of gifts to share, give a way, teach and bless you guy's with and now that I'm rested, I will be able to do just that.

Faith without works is dead and if I was out here claiming faith and not showing it, I was basically a zombie anyways so, what reason would I have to still be here on this earth taking up oxygen that could be used by somebody who is willing and able to do the work! I wouldn't have any valid reason.

Let's see, I sing, I write, I play, I compose, I'm a poet, songwriter, vocalist, author, play-write, entertainer, master of ceremonies, I'm funny, I'm a promoter, manager not to mention a few other things and I was not doing what I could to be that blessing that I ask to be daily. Do you know how many of you and others could be missing out on just because of my neglect? How many souls and or lives that could've possibly have been saved had I been more diligent? Well, I've been given another chance and I will not botch this one I promise you!

This book is the beginning along with some songs that have already been put on the market. I'm starting on my second book this week about growing up in the "Emerald Street Boys" rap group. I was in it as a teenager. I think it's something that needs to be talked about also, maybe something I need to get off my chest.

"All That Glitters Is Not Gold" the title.

I'm not sure how long it will take to complete this book because I'm going to take my time on this one.

Sugar Bear, Capt'n Crunch, Sweet- J — The Emerald Street Boy's

Edward Wells Jr (rip) Dr. James Croone Thatguy Rcurtis Jamerson

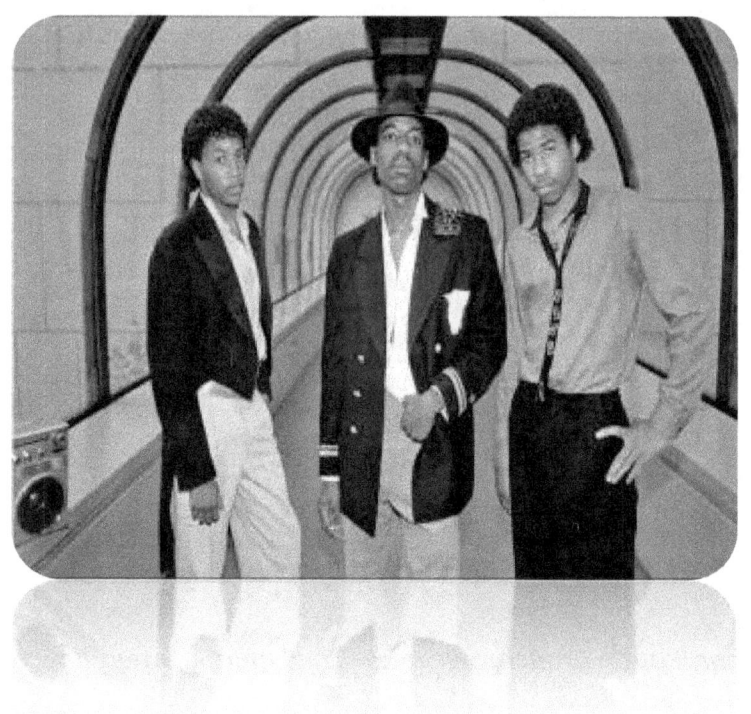

I was just saying to a friend of mine yesterday how as a kid you obtain valuable information that at that time you think is "hogwash" then once you start to mature you realize that you did retain that information and you can now use it in your daily life and activities.

That's the thing about the common sense we all have and seldom use. It's readily available to us though and it's good for our mental growth too. Imagine knowing something in your mind and spirit and still not utilizing it would that make any sense? No, it would not.

There are many of our brothers and sisters who fumble through their lives that way. Why? It is so much easier and peaceful to use what you got to get what you need and want. We're not supposed to be working hard, we should be working smart, we're not supposed to be struggling, we should be smiling while we prosper.

It has taken me 54 years to figure out much of this information I'm passing along to you right now in this book. That's 15 years more than it took the people of Egypt to stop walking in circles. It's a little sad in a way because I could've been helping way more people had I gotten it sooner. Everything has its time and place, season and reason, so I'm good with it. "Better now then never" right? Absolutely!

Isn't this a beautiful sight, doesn't it just make you feel like there is a higher power?

This has me missing being on a boat cruise; I love the water!

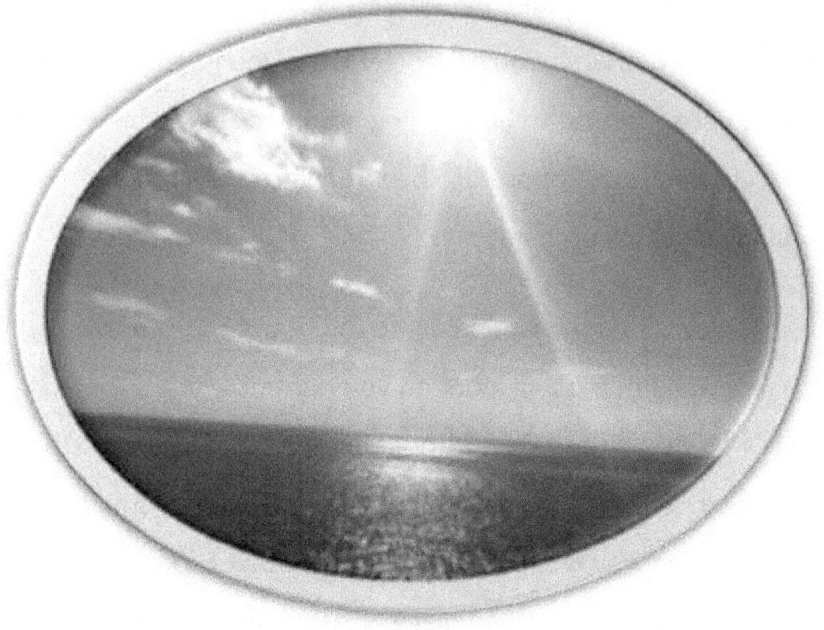

This is me in the Cayman Islands back in 2016. I Love it! It didn't matter about the other people on the boat I was determined to have a great time!

This was me away from the rest of my day-to-day living, shame on me if I didn't take advantage of it! So, I did take full advantage of it! Too bad I do not feel comfortable taking a cruise now. Oh well, maybe again, one day.

Sometimes we don't take the time to enjoy our own selves and for that reason there remains a void in our spirits because we are supposed to love ourselves first after God. How else can you spread love or love someone if you don't first love you? This life is short and we don't know how short it is until we're lifeless so, enjoy you! You're working to live not the other way around. There is a "HUGEMONGEST" world out there for

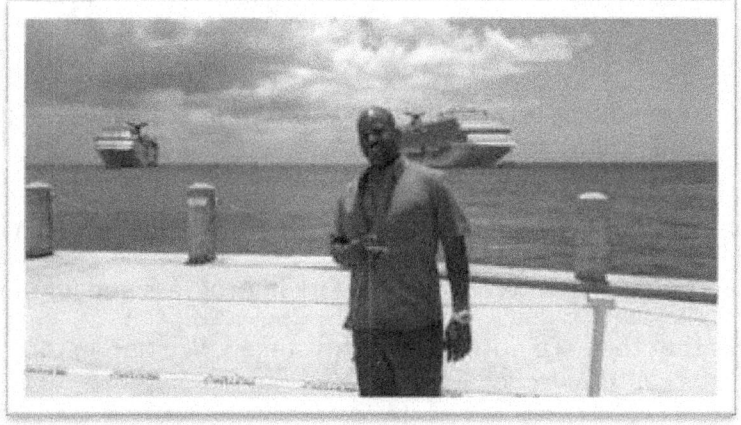

us to partake in the only thing that's stopping you is you. If you want to travel; travel, if you want to build a treehouse; build a treehouse, whatever you want to do for you do it! It's your right and you reserve it let know one tell you otherwise or convince you otherwise or you will be sorry and saddened.

This is important information to pass on to our youth or they'll be lost and confused just like most of them already are today. Every day that goes by and you have not made any forward progress is a wasted day. Try not to waste a day. Plan, write down your day's agenda on a piece of paper and as you accomplish each individual item of the day, scratch it off you will notice how much more you get done in a day, mind you I said write it down no input it on your computer or phone, write it down with paper and a pen or pencil it'll be more effective that way because you physically put in the work to refer to all day.

Am I doing this every day? No, why not? Because like you I'm human and I slip up. I do attempt too though. You know how it goes when it's tough to take your own advice you can certainly give it. We are all a work in progress and whoever thinks that they are not, are sadly mistaken. We don't stop growing and learning until we're "pushing up daisies" that's what we all need to comprehend.

I thank God for my mistakes and tough times because I realize that is where my growth comes from, my wisdom comes from the mistakes you make, and I learn from.

The day we decide we know everything is the day we need counseling.

I for one do not want to know everything, that is too much responsibility and I'm good.

Having this virus and going through the recovery process has been an experience I will never forget, and I will always respect. Almost sixty days and I'm still not fully healed. I'm just thankful that my brain wasn't affected while I was lacking oxygen and I'm thankful that my failed kidneys didn't rupture permanently. See, my God is sufficient, and he told me before I went through this that "he got me" I believed him and trusted him and look at me now, testifying and praising!

I'm not ashamed, afraid, embarrassed or anything like that because when it comes to my relationship with my father in heaven, it's second to none!

Second chances in this life are not to be taken lightly. Do your work diligently and without resentment and be a good son or daughter in the eyes of the lord.

Don't let your second chance be in vain too.

Make your mark in this crazy world as one of the ones who made something happen.

There are enough people making noise with their complaints and there should 'a, would 'a, could 'a. It's not easy to get started on a task; however, once you get momentum, it gets easier than you thought it could ever be. The hardest part is getting started. So, write down your plan of attack and by seeing it you'll then assert action. I find that we are creatures of habit therefore once we do something the same about 21 times or so, it becomes a habit. Something I learned some time back and I kept locked in.

Yesterday, I did something really stupid on my part and thankfully I live to tell the story. So, since my bout with Covid and my recovery I have not smoked any weed. Two nights ago, I thought I'd roll me one and it wouldn't light, or it would light, and not stay lit. Natasha said, that's God and thanked him. So yesterday I decided to have a THC drink with my brunch. Oh boy, was that a mistake! I'm thinking, no big deal I'm eating so, I should be just fine. Natasha comes downstairs and notices what I'm drinking and say's; "you're only supposed to have a shot of this!" Well, I was feeling cool until about a half an hour later. Shakes, head spinning, felt like I was never going to come down off this high, my mind was thinking and reflecting about everything I'd gone through in my whole entire life. It was crazy! Uh oh!

Change the subject!

It's that time of year again. That time of year that we are superficially generous to one another. We charge up our credit cards to the limit and then pay them back with our tax return monies. The time that we've chosen to take away the true meaning of and make it a "retail holiday" instead of a "thankful" holiday. The things we do as humans and God just overlooks.

Imagine, you sacrificed your son for your community and instead of your community acknowledging that day as a dedication of that sacrifice, they recognize it as something totally different and irrelevant. How would that make you feel? Don't answer, just think about it and then you may be able to appreciate God and his mercy and grace for us all. I myself, knowing me would not have any understanding and would act out! The nerve and the mitigated gall to oust the savior for a fat white man in a red suit and his elves. Lol, that doesn't even sound right! It sounds made up!

As if someone was hiding some truth!

As we journey through this life, we will find things out along the way that will have us feeling a little confused, shocked, amazed and enlightened all at the same time. That is when we are taking on more wisdom. Short time, we have to get what we can and spread it as we do. It is important and very necessary so, do your part and be rewarded ten-fold! Don't wait for it and make sure you're not doing it for the sole purpose of the reward you will be receiving. Do it because you're supposed to and out of a relationship. Blessings befall us every second of the day, we just don't recognize them as blessings. We take them for granted due to the fact of them not being big, expensive, mind blowing etc. We are too materialistic (me included) and it's because of society and their judgmental ways.

Don't wear white after the summer season..., Huhn? Who are you to tell me what to wear and when to wear it? If I ever let them, society and the judgmental people around me be the boss of me, check my temperature. Forget that! I will wear what I want when I want! That's the prophecy of a leader!

God has dominion over you and me, and that is it, period!

I know, I know, that seems to be all I talk about, right? Well, what else is there to talk about really? Don't answer that either. There is a lot we can discuss; however, without God, we have and are nothing!

We are coming to the end of this conversation about my experience with Covid and what I've gone through while dealing with the evil diabolical disease. I have a lot to be thankful for. I am alive, my health is better, and my love life is exceptional!

My football team is sucking in a major way though (Seahawks) I think we need a new coach because Pete is too old and set in his ways. I think Pete doesn't trust his quarterback enough to make his own calls. Plus, our offense of line has been horrible for quite a few years; don't understand that at all.

We might have to start from scratch, build a team with a new coach. This is just my opinion.

Unless Pete gets a little more aggressive, creative and starts using his players according to their talents and expertise.

Ok, I'm off the Seahawks now.

It's Monday and I feel great! I'm rejuvenated and my mind is clear. Mondays are usually a drag for most people. Mondays aren't a drag for me, I see it as another opportunity to get back on task and get things done. Businesses are now open for the week making it possible to accomplish most goals and pay bills. I know there are a lot of you that are letting your bills be paid by your financial institution, not me though I trust me, myself and I with the distribution of my funds! I bet the lot of you don't even balance your checkbook (so to speak) anymore and that's how we used to catch the banks stealing our money! We better get a little wiser and pay closer attention to this convenient thing we're falling for. Convenience is designed for lazy people to take short-cuts which allows sneaky, underhanded people to take full advantage of their chance to steal from you or take whatever they want.

These days it's so easy to slip up due to convenience, work smart and strong! Suck a's will test your patience level and convince you to stoop to their stupidity. Don't do it! You have way too much to lose, and they don't.

The amazing thing is how battling and recovering from Covid brought all this out in me. See, I told y'all I just needed rest in order to reach you with this information, information you would have never gotten if I never got that rest. There are a couple different ways to look at your challenging times; positively or negatively. I choose the first way only because it helps me stay on task and keeps me motivated. I also pass this information on to my children and grandchildren. I wake up. I thank God I send a motivational message to my children and grandchildren then my day begins. I think it's important for us to pass information within your home first then spread it elsewhere and, since home is where the heart is, that seems self-explanatory to me; start with your immediate family. Now, bear in mind that, sometimes the message received is just for you and not to be shared. Therefore, pray and ask for divine guidance so as not to disrupt a person or person's path with information you should have kept to yourself; it's a fine line between a blessing and a curse and, we are not equipped to determine that line folks! So, don't even take the chance.

Two nights ago, Natasha and I were driving to pick up some Pho and while we were almost at the restaurant, I noticed this guy pushing a cart full of everything he owned. It was raining and cold and all he had on was this little windbreaker type jacket. I told Natasha to pull over. I want to give him this leather coat in my trunk. I had this coat in my trunk for a couple of months meaning to drop it off at a clothing bin.

Well, we pulled over and I asked him if he wanted this coat I have in my trunk, and he said, "yes, all I have is this dollar my friend gave me." This man is homeless, and he was still willing to pay for the coat! Wow! Anyway, I gave him the coat and I told him that will keep him warm because it is well insulated. It was so funny because he was like, "hell yeah!" I said God bless and happy holidays he repeated the same and we went to pick up her Pho.

We never know when it's time to be a blessing until the time presents itself. I just felt it in my spirit to give this man that coat. I had good intentions for the coat already, God had better intentions though, and that is why that leather coat had been in my car for so long. The thing about God is..., he plans everything as it going to be, and it fits like a glove. Case and point, when that man put that leather coat on, it fit him like it was, tailor-made for him. I'm not telling you this for "attaboy" . I'm giving you this information so that you can perhaps feel a little different about less-fortunate people than yourself and be a blessing knowing that all you have is, Gods anyway. Meaning anytime…, he can take it away. Amen.

So, now there is a much worst Covid virus it's so much stronger that it has its own name. Why do they make these viruses and then let them loose on the humans across the universe? I mean, it's so evil and diabolical! Can be only the enemy and his demons.

Don't fall for the "okey-doke", this is real, these diseases are designed to kill us people!

And we also need to start getting along more. Together we're strong, divided we're vulnerable. Our sole purpose as a one people is to help each other and be examples to our youth. So far, our examples have failed!

Take heed and change! The change will manifest a new look on your life; you will be pleased my brothers and sisters.

Testimony time:

Since I've been recovering and even while I was suffering from the Covid, I have not been in need of anything. My bills did not fall behind, my home wasn't in jeopardy, my finances were actually increased! All because God told me, "I got you." And I believed him with no doubt. I mean I was making more money than my take home pay from my job! Are you serious?! Y'all need to get hip! He is real and he will see you through all your trials and tribulations if you trust him to do so.

Not only that, my placement at my place of employment is still there for me!!!

How many of you can testify to that? If that is not an awesome and faithful God, I don't know what is.

EVERYTHING IN MY LIFE WHILE I WAS UNABLE TO STAND ON MY TWO FEET, WAS TAKEN CARE OF!!!

I'm not bragging to you guys, I'm testifying and confessing and trying to wake some of y'all up to the goodness and the promise of God..., he's not a man so, he can't lie. When he tells you something, count it done! Now, it will not be in your time it will be in his time which is always, "on time" he is never late with his promises.

People!!!!!!!

If what you're doing is not working, then try something that has been tried and proven since the day of time; a relationship with the "most high" seriously, because if it doesn't work, you can always go back to your old ways.

Okay, I've testified and confessed and now it's time to finish the book.

Who fights for their life and decides to author a book while doing so? Me, that's who. When my spirit speaks to me, I answer and conform. When my soul gives me an order, it's done, period.

This is why you are now reading these words in this book. So, thank you for your support!

You know what? I only wanted to be a musician, singer, songwriter, producer, promoter and entertainer. Now, I'm an author, talk show host and motivator. We can plan our own way, that does not mean it will come to pass. Life has its own agenda and if you don't know how to adjust, (oh boy) you are in for a very bumpy road!

I wanted to have a mortgage by now unfortunately, I got sick and was unable to complete that goal. Now, there is a bubble that is soon to burst in real estate and next year is going to be a better time to purchase a home or homes. If I didn't know how to adjust and accentuate the positive, I'd be lost right now.

I'm glad that I went through what I went through in order to get to where I'm at. Growth mentally, physically, emotionally, and spiritually is important and that is why I say I'm glad I went through all that I did.

As long as I have breath in my body my life will have meaning and I will be a blessing. I will lead and not follow the ones who are leading us into the "gates of hell." It's the time to "man-up!" we are our only hope, and we need to realize that.

All races, all colors, all creeds, all religions, all people! Everyone! Everyone! ALL PEOPLE!

This shit is not easy, let me tell you. Recovering from a disease that could have easily taken my life is hard. Lungs have to be repaired. I have to get used to not being able to do all of the things I used to do before Covid and, it really sucks! I want to lift weights and do my push-ups like I used to do. I want to hang out and go sing with the bands like I used to do. I want to be as active as I used to be. I can't think about it, at least not right now. I know I need to just be thankful to be alive and I am, I just want to be freer to be and do. I've talked to folks who had it in the early stages of the outbreak and a year plus later, they still have residual complications they're dealing with. So., I know I'm damned lucky! I have been trying to record some songs and work with the voice a little and it's not hard. I just have to adjust to my range now as opposed to before.

Wrote a song for my fiancé called "God Hand Picked 4me" . She likes it, said that it's my real R&B song, and she said it's much more different from any of the song's I've written. That made me feel good because I wanted it to be more soulful and pretty; I achieved that goal. I think my pinky finger on my left hand is finally starting to show some signs of waking up, it's not as numb as it normally is and, I love that! It was a weird feeling to have constantly. I now have a pain in my hip that comes and goes whenever it deems necessary. My physical therapist thinks that it's because of our routines getting more challenging for my body. Ok, I'll take that. Weights, medicine balls have been added to our work-out sessions. I'm amazed at how simple body movement can be so tough, I mean bouncing the medicine ball, stepping up on a platform about a foot and a half with twenty-five pounds in each hand and things of that nature; sort of tough. I'm going hard at it though because I want my life back!

Every day is starting to be more challenging as well because It's seeming like I'm running out of things to do to keep my brain motivated. I guess I should be working on "Thatguy Rcurtis Show " making sure I have a guest scheduled for the next season. I think I'm getting a little restless and complacent. I don't mean to; I'm just noticing it. I've got to get back to writing down my agenda and sticking to the plan! It's crazy because it has only been three months and I'm already slowing down. One thing I haven't slowed down with is, praying every day and thanking God for everything. I don't anticipate that changing any time soon or ever! Like I said I am attempting to record, and my physical therapist told me that is good for my lung training. I am on social media seeing (vocalists old and new) singing at these open mics and with their own bands and I am wishing I could perform. All in due time and, I get that, no seriously, I do, I'm just super ready mentally and passionately to get back in the game; physically..., nope! – Choices E40!

I'm ready to do what I do best, disrupt the game and give it a new approach. I will be performing live for the first time in years. I was asked to do a repast for one of the mothers of the community who recently got her wings. I jumped at the chance because I was honored to be considered. I will have a three- or four-piece band and it's going to be very entertaining and groovy! I cannot wait. I will be playing the drums and singing. It will be challenging; I'm up for the challenge. This recovery time has been good for me, I've gotten much better at drumming and my coordination has improved tremendously! This will be a show that will be talked about and remembered!

It's forcing me to try something I've never attempted before, virtual band rehearsal! With our current conditions and the fact that it is not getting any better any time soon I must be creative and forth-right. I'm excited!

I know a person who has had the virus twice! The first time was when it hit us in two thousand, the second was after he was vaccinated and after he got his booster shot as well; my son also attracted Covid after his vaccination. Neither one of them were bad off, just a few minor symptoms; headache, mild cough and things like that. I'm not sharing this information with you to discourage you from getting vaccinated or anything of that nature, no I'm just sharing information with you. Everything is not for everybody; I truly believe that our spirits will lead us to what is meant for us as individuals. I myself, having been down with the virus, still possess the antibodies and will still have a positive covid test if I were to take it right now so, I'm not safe unless I practice being safe; masking up, staying home unless it's necessary to go out etc.

This Covid thing has really taken a toll on my body. My breathing isn't the same even after four months of recovery, I must learn how to regulate my breathing based on my activity. Considering the alternative though…, I'm cool! I have no complaints, I am blessed to be alive, I am thankful for a second chance at this thing called life, I am ecstatic to be able to be a part of my grandbaby's lives, I do appreciate the fact that my finances were blessed in abundance while I am recuperating, I did thoroughly enjoy my Christmas celebration this year and I am looking forward to the future ahead of me! God is good!

I can honestly say that my happiness within me is being enhanced daily due to a family who welcomed me with open arms and no expectations, my relationship with my siblings (the ones that want to be in a relationship) and the love my grown children show to me. It's awesome!!!

My experience with Covid has opened my eyes to a lot of good things and I'm thankful for it!

My relationship with God is the best it's ever been, simply because I am now giving him his time.

My attitude is no nonsense and, at the same time, patient. I feel like there is nothing I can't do as long as I put God ahead of it all, seriously! I feel like this is my time to show and not tell.

This is the time to not let anyone take you off your motivated mission, it's the time to focus and make things happen!

No complaining, no giving up, no giving into frustration, no holding your head down, no "passing the buck" just plain ol' handle your business, then watch your stock exceed more than you thought possible!

And, with God anything is possible!

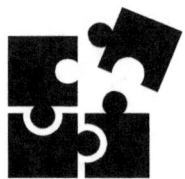

CHAPTER SEVENTEEN

Woke up this morning to another associate hospitalized with the evil disease Covid. I could tell he was a little scared because he was on social media asking for prayer and you could see it in his eyes. I sent him a message telling him to not allow his head to take over. I told him to rely on his faith. I told him God is in control. I told him if he let his head take over, he would not make it out of the hospital. I let him know that I too had gone through and was hospitalized for three weeks.

People, you cannot comprehend unless you have gone through the whole ordeal, it is no fun! I can scare you literally to death! Faith is of the utmost importance in this situation; I can't stress it enough.

So far this week, there have been three people that I know of that have been stricken by this evil disease Covid.

Y'all better be careful out there, better keep them mask on regardless of you being vaccinated or not!

They have so many variances now that they are not even sure if the damned vaccine will continue to work anymore!

I was watching a television show about Nelson Mandela's grandson and his movement. It seems that he is still concerned about HIV/AIDS and he's campaigning for a cure. That got me thinking about how that was the topic of all discussions and now you barely hear about it and there are still millions of people dying from it.

Why did we just dismiss this subject and neglect anymore care for its cure?

Interesting, isn't it? I think so.

Why does the power -to -be, choose what is important and what is not important or not important anymore? Where is the fairness there? There is no fairness, life isn't fair. That is why we literally have to make our own way and choose our own path to leave a trail with. Leaders are needed now more than ever, follower's coma a dime a dozen and unless they're following the right leaders..., they are just in the way. Intelligent human beings are under-rated. I'm talking about the ones we consider squares, nerds, weirdo's and any other derogatory term we can come up with.

They are the humans that utilize more than ten percent of their brain, they are the humans who work off of common sense not normalcy. They are not afraid of being alone with their thoughts, they embrace it and grow smarter and wiser. They do have faith in God, they do know that without him they would not exist. They are you and me as well as our friends and relatives if we stop and think before making our next move. I know that may have flown way up over your heads; however, if you reach up high enough, it'll still be there for you to capture and keep.

Bottom line, think before you speak, only talk if you have something prevalent or at least relevant to say, listen more than you talk, wait before you react that way you can now respond, SHUT UP sometimes and learn something new. Words for the wise.

You know how we seldom take our own advice; well, I think I'm beyond that currently in my life because I pray for divine guidance and wisdom therefore affording me the mind to listen more and wait a little longer.

We never know what is in us until we must perform or release it. For example, one time while being incarcerated for a week I fasted for that entire week: no water, no food, just prayer, bible and push-ups.

Now, I know we've been taught that we can't go without water, and I don't know for how long "they" say.

Ok, according to Wikipedia, a human being can survive three to five days without the intake of water. So, according to them I was right at my threshold. I didn't know this at that time, I just knew my God and trusted in him. I didn't care about what the masses said about it, I just did based on my faith. As a kid, I was chased by a dog, and I jumped over a fence to get away. I had no fear of not making that jump, I just knew I was going to not get bit or eaten by that vicious dog. I'm saying this to reiterate how we don't know what we can do until we must do what we must do to survive.

I have been home for four months now and I am ready to get back to business. I can't go back at eighty percent, if I'm not a hundred percent I am no good to the company or more importantly, myself. So, I have been taking it easy and slow following doctors orders and being obedient to my body. I tell you guys what, if I never have to go through something like this again, it'll be too soon! I wouldn't wish this on my first or last enemy ever!

It's terrible you guys!

I'm ready I believe I said this earlier; I'm shooting for the second or third week in January 2022. That's my goal.

I have been asked to perform for a repass. For those of you who don't know what a repass is, it's the celebration of the home going for your loved one who has transitioned to their paradise.

So, I was honored because it is for one of the matriarchs of my community growing up. So, I will be playing drums and singing along with a bass player, keyboardist and possibly a guitarist and trumpeter. This is going to be my biggest challenge yet; I mean after the recovery. I've been working on my chops and focusing on my pocket. To me pocket is the most important position for a drummer, after all we are the rhythm for the groove.

We will play a few more instrumentals than usual so that I can pace myself singing. I'm really excited about it though!

This is like a dream come true for me. As a kid my plan was to sing and perform, produce and finally, be a drummer in a jazz band. Well. This is not a jazz band per-say I am still playing the drums in the band the singing while playing wasn't exactly in the original plans. "We never know what we can do, right?"

My friends are about to figure out what to do on January 6, 2022.

I think I will probably do more shows as my lungs permit. My passion is music always has been and always will be,

Starting with a benefit recovery concert performance sometime next year, mandatory masks throughout the whole concert performance. Now that is going to take some creativity to convince the attendees to conform to this concert mandate again, "we never know what we can do" right?

This is going to be an awesome performance and concert! Will probably be the best performance of all my performances!

A benefit concert for Covid survivors: I had Covid And, I survived the concert.

Big plans for 2022 and beyond! Once I'm fully recovered; no stopping me from my path! I will have gotten the rest I needed to continue my journey for hope, prosperity and choices!

The New year will be here in three days. 3, 2, 1...

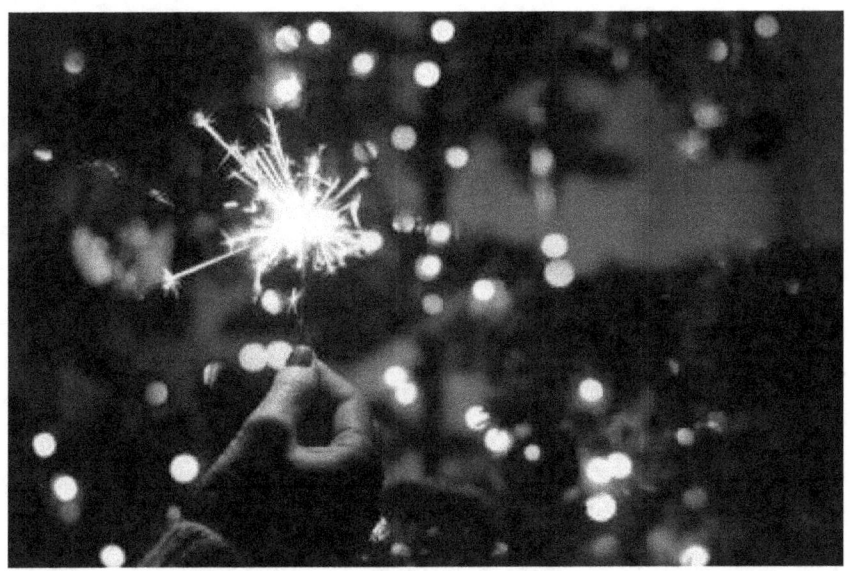

Well, the new year is here! I spoke with my son at midnight as well as my daughter, granddaughter and grandson. We brought in the new year in the safe in the comforts of our home. It was great! We toasted our family, a prosperous and fun filled two thousand twenty-two and then of course I thanked my God for another year. This is the year of accomplishments and being a major blessing to many. I'm excited! This is the year I got married to the most wonderful woman that I could've ever had the opportunity to meet last year. We will be a power couple for all and many to be inspired by.

All this time without doing the math, I thought I was 23 when my daughter was born until last night. We figured out that I was 22 years old. Now, check this out. I was 22 years of age when I had my daughter who was a definite blessing for me and, this year 2022 I will be marrying my latest "hand – picked" blessing on the 22nd of April.

Awesome!

My life is getting better and better on a daily basis just like my recovery and it feels good.

I've noticed here lately that I am the best man that I've ever been and it's all due to the rest I got while dealing with Covid and the recovery. I was told last night that I have (definitely) matured and grown in this short time of them knowing me. I really appreciated that comment because it wasn't expected nor was there any malice behind it. When they said it, I felt it coming from their soul and good spirit. So, I thanked them and let them know that I knew where the comment came from within them. I felt like that was important for me to relay to them, that way they would know that I felt them and was honored that they would drop a gem like that on me randomly.

People often do not take the time to appreciate one another, they just keep it moving like a compliment or an acknowledgement is going to kill them. Huge problem in our society these days. So, I make sure you know, I appreciate you when necessary.

We have got to do better you guys; kindness is not out of style.

So, two thousand twenty -two who knew we'd make it to this point? Got some news today via Facebook that one of my musician comrades didn't make it. Incredible keyboardist and drummer, "D". I remember the first time I saw him play the drums, I forget where we were at the time all I know is I was impressed, I approached him about joining my band at the time and he obliged me; I believe the band was called "Gravy" anyway, "D" was always late and always showed up with a box of wine (for himself). Good dude though, easy going sweet spirited brotha. He'll be missed in the music community for sure. Another one gone too soon, Lady "D"; a drummer that always wore a smile and had a kind word. You two rest in heavenly peace.

We never know when our time on this earth will expire, that is why it is important to have your relationship tight and right with God, in my humble opinion. It's one thing to die, it's another thing to die and not know where you are going afterwards. Not to say you know for sure; however, at least you'll have a good idea because of your relationship with the almighty.

Omicron, the new Covid. Just like the Devil this virus is sneaky and conniving; the symptoms you may have, or you may not have and, if you are vaccinated and boosted..., you become A- symptomatic! Wow, you become a carrier of the virus not to mention this one is airborne as well. What's next? Never mind, I don't want to know. Nuclear weapons, biochemical weapons, man is just ushering in the enemy daily. Inviting evil into our bloodstream, mind, body, and spiritual existence without even knowing it. Bamboozled! Man, thinks the Devil doesn't exist, like all these stupid decisions belong to him, man really thinks he's that intelligent! I am cracking up right now as I write this because how could he feel that way when he himself says, we only use ten percent of our brain? Now, you're probably cracking up too because those two scenarios don't equate. Anyhow, I am on a rampage for souls being saved because although I know it's not possible, it would be great if we all landed in heaven after it's all said and done. I will do my part to show you what having a relationship with God and walking in your blessing will do for you. And that's my word which I break for no one!

When finances are not threatened you feel a whole lot better about your day-to-day, it's a more secure feeling when you don't have to worry about your bills. That is a security every one of us is after. Prayer then your works will have you there. Like I said in the beginning of this book, I will be speaking about my relationship with God a lot in this book because without him I would not exist, nor would I be, the who, I am. Just to let you know, I am not trying to convince you of anything as far as being a believer; just testifying and relaying my experience with you is all. Now, should this help one of you, then none of these words are in vain.

ABOUT THE AUTHOR

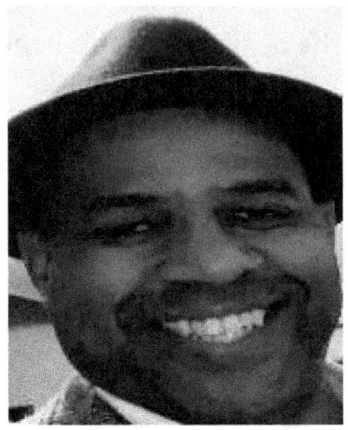

Rcurtis Fantpayne Jamerson is singer, songwriter, musician, performer, car salesperson, talk show host, emcee, promoter, father, grandfather and highly active and healthy normally. Born and raised in Seattle Washington except for three years in Los Angeles California. Pretty laid back and stays out the way on purpose. Music and performing is the real passion! Being a part of the first rap group to get some notoriety in Seattle (The Emerald Street Boys) it allowed for a little local fame (if you will) you can see them in "The Northwest Passage" at the (EMP) Experience Music Project along with Sir Mix-a-lot and a few others. Check out "Thatguy Rcurtis Show" (formally RnR Live Jamm Session Presents) he started back in March 2020 when musicians and their fans could no longer hang together so, he produced a way they could at least stay in touch. Now, the show has evolved into a platform with such guest; entrepreneur's, business owners, doctors, scientist, music producers, and just successful people willing to speak about their journey to their goal and it his hope that it motivates the audience to go for their own dreams. At the end of the day, Rcurtis just wants to be a blessing to as many people as he can. While in the hospital battling with Covid he noticed that there was a need for a book to talk about the experience so, he was inspired to write it instead of waiting on the virus to either take him or let him go, he started writing. Thus, "I Had Covid And, It Hurt's" was born. Enjoy, mask-up and God bless.

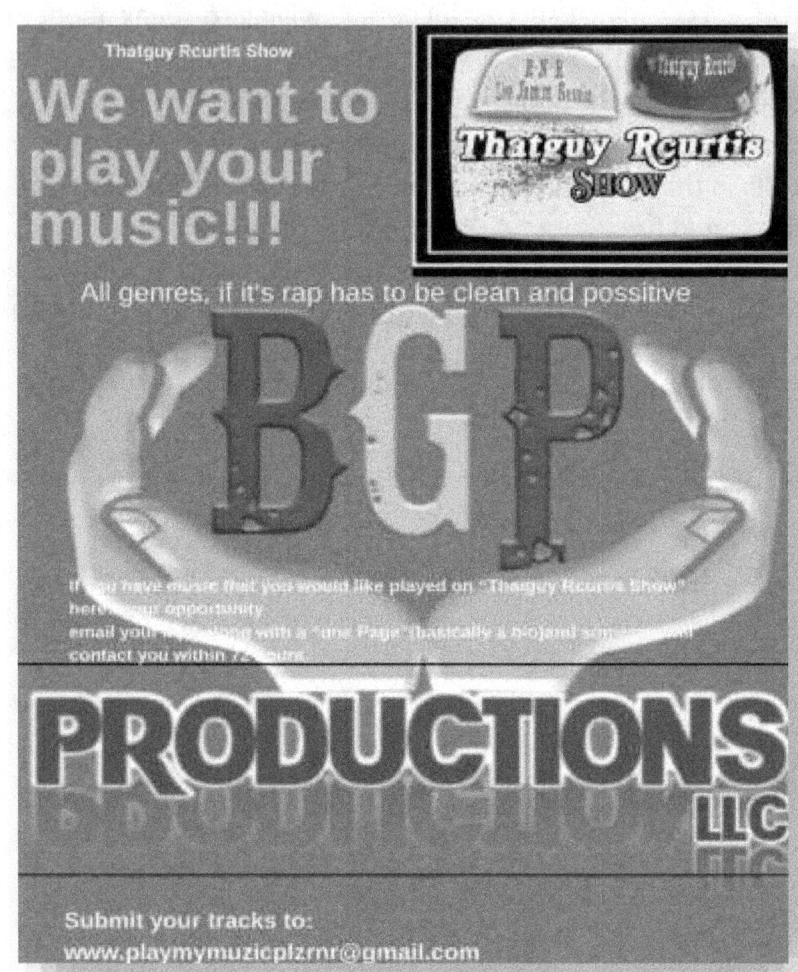

www.ingramcontent.com/pod-product-compliance
Lightning Source LLC
Chambersburg PA
CBHW072147290526
45794CB00004B/1436